AT THE WAY WE DO HEALTH-CARE
IN AMERICA

IF YOU THINK HEALTH-CARE IS UNAFFORDABLE NOW...

WAIT TILL IT'S FREE

THE PLAGUE OF SOCIALIZED MEDICINE AND THE ONLY KNOWN CURE.

COLIN GUNN AND
DR. PHILIP R. OLSSON

Published by Gunn Productions LLC, Waco, Texas.

ISBN: 978-1514332504

More information about the *Wait Till It's Free* film: www.WTIFree.com
More information about Gunn Productions LLC: www.ColinGunn.com

Cover Artist: Austin Collins
Layout Artist: Zyrek Castelino

TABLE OF CONTENTS

ACKNOWLEDGEMENTS

We wish to thank those who had a hand in the production of this little companion volume.

Undoubtedly, to whatever extent the enclosed chapters educate or motivate readers to see health-care in the U.S. with new eyes, the Real People featured in Wait Till It's Free deserve much credit for that. The cast includes Steven Brill, Tim Carney, Tony Dale, Theodore Dalrymple, Juliette Madrigal-Dersch (MD), Kyle Duncan, Alieta Eck (MD), Daniel Hannan, Tom Kendall (MD), John Mackey, Jane Orient (MD), Ron Paul, Patrick Pullicino (MD), Andrew Schlafly, Phyllis Schlafly, Keith Smith (MD), and Scott Stoll (MD). These and several others each contributed to the message and movement of both the film and this book.

Many thanks to those who reviewed chapters or larger sections of the text and suggested concrete improvements: Adam Brink, Dr. Richard Edgerly, Emily Gunn, Brooke Kaczor, and Jason Storms. Joining their number later in the writing process, Pieter Friedrich unsheathed the editorial equivalent of a surgeon's scalpel and helpfully carved up many a sentence, bringing happy results. A hearty thanks, of course, goes out to Austin Collins, owner and design lead at My Hero Media, for constructing a colorful and engaging cover.

We appreciate the support of Samaritan Ministries International for this project and the generous and proactive members of the Association of American Physicians and Surgeons (AAPS), many of whom took time out of their schedules to grant extended interviews to a certain Scottish Texan and his filmmaking crew.

Lastly, we say thanks to our families, the Gunn and Olsson clans respectively. Thank the Lord, first, for the gift of a godly wife. Emily Gunn and Heather Olsson, thank you for bearing with us and for bearing in great quantity and quality our covenant children. Naturally, we will name them, starting with the Gunns: Grace, Noah, Knox, Molly, Mercy, Patience, Charity, Stedfast, and Theodore. Now the Olssons (at least those still at home): Joseph, Gabrielle, and Cora. You are each a precious gift, fashioned by our True Physician and Deliverer of New Rewards.

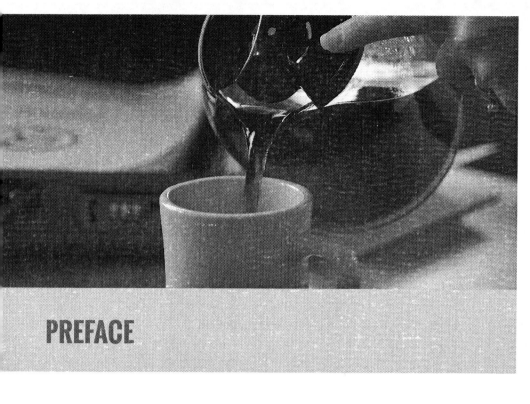

PREFACE

> Health care is too expensive, so the Clinton administration is putting a high-powered corporate lawyer in charge of making it cheaper. (This is what I always do when I want to spend less money-hire a lawyer from Yale.) If you think health care is expensive now, wait until you see what it costs when it's free.
>
> PJ. O'ROURKE

It was over twenty years ago that P.J. O'Rourke delivered that line at a gala dinner celebrating the opening of the Cato Institute's new headquarters in D.C. No doubt it was many dozens of lawyers ago and thousands of unreadable (or at least unread) pages of health-care "reform" legislation ago too.

Some things don't change. In addition to Washington's surplus of lawyers and unread bills, one of the things that don't change is human economic behavior. If you didn't learn in high school or home school economics the principle of TANSTAAFL, then you should give your teacher (mom?) a bit of a hard time about it. There Ain't No Such Thing As A Free Lunch. Even when lunch is offered at "zero price," eating it still comes with costs. For the consumer of the lunch, the cost is "opportunity cost"—i.e., what's given up to eat the lunch. For the supplier, the cost is what was required in financial and other mental and material resources to furnish the meal.[1]

Other than Jesus, humans lack the absolute ability to render scarce resources not-so-scarce. God can fry an egg by speaking. I cannot. Indeed, even when U.S. Treasury agents print or coin fiat currency (derived from the Latin "let it be done"), they're stuck using the paper and metal ultimately supplied by the real (Triune) lord of the universe. We humans are the recipients of creation and (some of us) of redemption absolutely FREE of charge. In his teachings about kingdom ethics in Matthew 5, Jesus reminds his hearers that the Father "makes his sun rise on the evil and on the good, and sends rain on the just and on the unjust." He also, in verses 27 through 30, reminds those who would be his disciples that their heavenly Father not only owns the cattle on a thousand hills but is capable of arranging them so as to benefit those who trust him:

> Which of you by worrying can add one cubit to his stature? So why do you worry about clothing? Consider the lilies of the field, how they grow; they neither toil nor spin; and yet I say to you that even Solomon in all his glory was not arrayed like one of these. Now if God so clothes the grass of the field, which today is, and tomorrow is thrown into the oven, will He not much more clothe you, O you of little faith.

The Lord is able to provide goods and services (e.g., angelic protection) out of His unlimited abundance. Whereas we must use the materials and conditions he provides, establishes, and sustains by his powerful Word.

Even so, though sunshine and rain are generally abundant (being of divine origin), humans do not have equal access even to those "commodities." Some people own more things than others or at least own things generally judged as higher quality. This helps to explain why not everyone lives on beachfront property in Malibu, California. Beachfront property in Malibu is in scarce supply and so is reserved, as the finer things tend to be,

---

1   For an entertaining and illustrative article about some basic economic concepts, see Dan Sanchez, https://www.mises.org/daily/6913/How-Saving-Grows-the-Economy; Internet; 10 October 2014.

for the higher bidders. This is where the matter of health-care provision enters the picture.

Especially due to the advances of science and markets within Western Civilization over the past two centuries, the beachfront property of high quality and often heroic medical care has become increasingly available to a greater proportion of the planet. Truly, the monetary cost could be far greater for much of what medical science and technology offer us. We are indeed materially blessed in astounding and innumerable ways.

There have been disturbing trends, however, for many years in the direction of higher health-care costs. This doesn't seem right, if we assume that genuinely free markets generally produce higher quality products and services for increasingly lower costs to consumers. While I grant that it may not address all the reasons for higher costs, an important part of our response to the inflationary trends must include the observation that if anything is scarce over the past 50 years it's a genuinely free market in health-care.

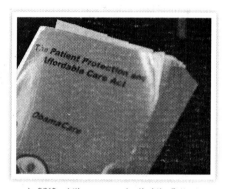

On March 23, 2010, President Barack Obama signed into law the Patient Protection and Affordable Care Act (or Affordable Care Act, or "Obamacare"). But that event and its aftermath, which

In 2010, a bill was passed called the Patient Protection and Affordable Care Act-otherwise known as Obamacare.

we're witnessing, should surprise no one. We can accustom ourselves to thinking about the heinous possible future being at least one bridge—as yet uncrossed—still in front of us. But while Obamacare has amounted to a significant bridge-crossing in itself, it is only the most recent (granted, it's a big bridge—rivaling that new one in San Francisco Bay) in a long series of worrisome warnings that precede crossings. And it's hard not to think that we are living in a place we warned ourselves about.

Yet this book does not aim merely to spin a tragic politico-economic tale. That reality is present. But another aim of the book is to reassure that there is hope for the restoration of economic sanity, improved (innovative) care, and a healthier, godlier population. In what follows, I attempt to expand the glimpse offered in the *Wait Till It's Free* documentary into both health-care woes and the reasons for hope and also to encourage deeper thinking and Christian meditation upon the topics raised.

It's my wish that the reader will find the jaunt through these pages to be entertaining and informative. It's also my prayer that together we will be moved toward greater faithfulness to God in how we think about and act with respect to health issues, how we care for the Body of Christ, and how we steward the resources entrusted to us by the Lord.

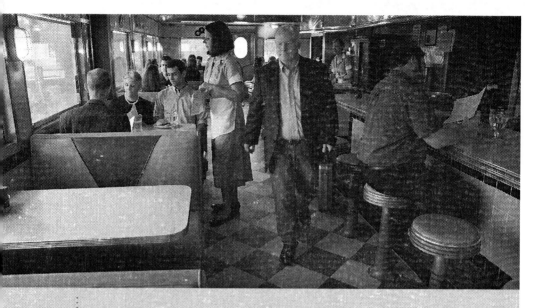

1 EXPECT THE UNEXPECTED

ENTERING THE DINER

In setting out to make *IndoctriNation*, my collaborators and I knew we needed a visual image to carry the narrative. Much more heavily than a piece of literature, a film depends on the use of strong visual images in order to establish themes, communicate ideas, and move the viewer to principled action. For that earlier film, we picked the imagery of the Big Yellow Bus to symbolize the centralized and impersonal character of government-controlled education. Like a clumsy yellow box on wheels, public schooling slogs down our streets and consumes our little ones throughout the day. As we thus set out to fashion a new film, we realized that the icon of the yellow bus served quite well in conveying the message of *IndoctriNation*.

What we needed now was an equally strong image to act as a unifying thread throughout *Wait Till It's Free*. But shots of hospital waiting rooms and surgery theaters are pretty common fare in films within the health-care documentary genre. And so a fresh, inspiring image or set of images was definitely in order for our film. But what?

In that search for a fresh inspiration, we hit upon the classic American diner as our centerpiece image.

I have always fantasized about sitting in a diner, chatting with lonely customers at the counter, and pestering the busy wait staff until late into the night. Hopper's "Nighthawks, 1942" painting, like many of his works, displays the loneliness of American life—a smattering of individuals congregating at the local corner joint. But to me the diner has always seemed like the place to be. Diners, in my mind, have a romantic (ok, perhaps a romantically lonely) character.

It was my love for that image and feeling of the old-fashioned American diner that led it to its taking center-stage in *Wait Till It's Free*. Unlike the looming, ubiquitous bus, however, the diner presents a positive image. It represents to me an America still boasting a vibrant immigrant population and recalls some of the better American values and symbols: choice, friendliness, mom and pop economics, endless cups of coffee, and, of course, apple pie. I also knew that this film needed to tell a clearly *American* story and the diner appeared second to none in helping to convey that.

Even beyond evoking nostalgia, however, the diner appeals to the economist in me. It serves to remind me how a number of small economic transactions (two genuine, copper pennies for a cup of coffee in 1942) can help create a bright, interesting, lively place—a place for people to cross paths. The diner was open and sometimes buzzing when nothing else was. It was often awake and playing host to conversation while the rest of town was snoozing.

Where it can still be found, a good diner offers a distinct kind of experience. You can usually find what you *expect* to find there. Art deco, shiny leather seats, spirited waitresses, burgers, fries, sodas, pies. In promising and delivering such charms, diners provide predictability and simplicity. Without too much trouble, you can know what's on the menu and what it's going to cost you.

A lively market is generally accompanied by a certain kind of predictability. In fact, predictability is a precondition for people acting in economically rational ways. Sadly, however, for anyone who's looked very closely, "predictable and orderly" hardly sums up our current health-care arrangements in America, least of all with the way that goods and services are priced. When prices are in persistent disarray, that's a sign that there are likely significant and repeated disruptions preventing the clear transmission of signals between various suppliers and consumers of goods and services. Picture a storm that's knocked out the traffic lights, creating stop-and-go traffic and sometimes even the occasional collision.

Let's return to the diner analogy for just a moment longer. Many who advocate for a "State as father (and father knows best)" approach to civil government protest any attempt to compare the provision of health-care goods and services to the provision of food. But these are the same people who, if they were forest rangers, would only be happy if all the trees were kept equal, by hatchet axe and saw. On another note, health-care goods and services are treated in their worldview somewhat like cows are treated in Hinduism. They are not only to be appreciated; they are to be reckoned as *sacred*. They are most definitely not something to be paired with lettuce, tomatoes, and a bun and sold for a buck fifty to a well-informed consumer swiveling at the counter.

But like the Hindus, these folks allow their religion (let's call it Statist Interventionism) to trump their better judgment. The activities of supplying and marketing food versus "health-care" are by no means radically different. Placed in the best possible light, the supply and consumption of both food and "health services" relates to the nourishing and caring for human bodies. Moreover, exchanges of those goods and services with the label "health-care" slapped on are not somehow magically exempted from the mundane realities of supply and demand.

An important goal of this book is to meditate on ways in which economic laws are displayed in the world of health-care and to see what happens (like a remorseful prophet pointing out the folly around him) when people attempt to "do" health-care in defiance of sound economic principles.

HUMAN NEEDINESS, CILANTRO, AND MEDICAL BILLING

A fundamental principle of economics we should all be able to agree on is this: human beings are 100% need. Any theologian worth his salt knows this. Any theologian worth his salt, therefore, is in immediate possession of a fundamental principle of economics. Humans (not to mention, all other creatures) are a needy lot.

We need air to breath, water to drink, and food to eat. We need to move our little bodies around, so our legs don't get blood clots and our midsections don't get too swollen. As individuals, we need others—human contact, mutual support, fellowship. Sometimes, through fault of our own, we need support in the form of medical aid because our dietary indiscretions, physical inactivity, substance abuse, sexual misdeeds, or other failures have taken a toll (i.e., the price one pays for going there.).

On top of that, human beings are everywhere confronted by risk and the fact of their own mortality. The question is generally not whether but when and how death will eventually occur for each of us (Heb. 9:27).[1]

At some point, not necessarily through fault of our own, we will each be smitten with disease or injury and require some professional intervention if we would remain well or, at least, alive. Thankfully, we are not all eager to speed our way toward the grave. Due to a lingering (though, in many places, waning) value that human communities place upon human life, as well as the many good inventions and innovations that make up modern medicine, we have inherited a revered concept of the person in need. We call this person "the patient."

Bottom line: we all face the prospect of being the patient at one time or another.

One gentleman I interviewed had fairly recently got a taste of this reality. Who would have guessed it would have a distinct cilantro flavor? But it did, according to Roger Stuber.

People like Roger make it pleasant to live among the humans. He's straightforward, friendly, and practical. A building contractor, he leaned against the exposed stud of an unfinished house and talked honestly and humorously about his experiences. He told me how several months earlier he started tasting cilantro in his mouth intermittently throughout the day. This experience persisted for some time.

Round about the same time, members of Roger's family began noticing that his usually very sound memory appeared to be slipping a bit. When I sat down with him and his wife, Gwen, she recalled that an automatic replay feature seemed to have developed in her husband's brain and that people were noticing and growing concerned:

> He would repeat stories and repeat stories and repeat stories…
> The kids and I just thought, "Well, maybe he's getting older

---

1   All biblical quotes are taken from the ESV, unless indicated otherwise.

and this is part of his aging process." But it became apparent to the kids and to myself and, also, the gentleman that he works with that this is more... than possible aging problems, that this is serious memory issues... I was talking with my older son, Jacob, and he said, "Mom, you really need to get him to a doctor and have him looked at because this is not normal." And I think when he said that to me I realized that this is something very serious and we need to get him some help.[2]

Shortly thereafter Roger made his way to a doctor's office.

After an MRI and some consultations with neurologists, Roger learned he had been having epileptic seizures and would require surgery. He had been suffering from something akin to a varicose vein—a cavernous venous malformation—in the right frontal lobe of his brain. A blood vessel had

become kinked and was leaking, causing the glitches in his memory and the funny cilantro-esque taste in his mouth.

Thank the Lord, the surgery to remove the kinked brain vein proved successful and Roger's cognitive functioning has since returned to normal.

But there was another taste left in Roger's mouth as a result of interfacing with the medical

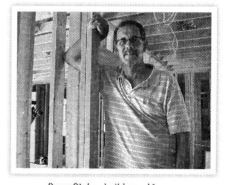

Roger Stuber, builder and former missionary pilot, gave us a close-up of his recent experience with medical billing.

establishment that is characteristic of American health-care. It related to the matter of billing. Roger didn't have health insurance and wasn't a government dependent. Consequently, he was inclined to be mindful of the costs incurred for his care.

In that vein (no pun intended), during the process of initially assessing his condition, Roger had an MRI scan of his brain. For that first scan, he was quoted $1,554. He subsequently underwent a second MRI, which was quoted at $5,222, almost quadruple the cost of the first. What's interesting

---

2   All quotes from individuals that are not hereafter footnoted are drawn directly from video interview footage that may or may not have made it into the *Wait Till It's Free* film.

is that he later learned that an insurer would have paid under $800 for the second of the two (for a reference, go to www.healthcarebluebook.com). But why such a discrepancy in price for the same services rendered, depending on whether the payer is an uninsured individual or an insurance company?

Here we begin to face the challenges encountered by cash-pay patients, those marginalized (i.e., uninsured or "under-insured") persons dwelling on the outskirts of a health-care system heavy laden with third-party involvement. Thankfully, Roger had going for him that he'd worked as a foreign missionary earlier in life and was accustomed to haggling in the marketplace. As a contractor, he also knew about negotiating from the standpoint of a service provider. Consequently, he at least was not as intimidated as a less savvy consumer might be when he received bills exceeding $70,000 for services rendered.

It wasn't, however, all about demonstrating some kind of "bargaining machismo." An important feature of this story relates to the fact that Roger belongs to a Christian health-care sharing ministry, in which the financial burdens incurred for medical needs are voluntarily shared through a direct financial support network. So when he went to negotiate bill reductions, he ranked high among his priorities the principle of acting as a wise steward of the dollars he would receive from individuals and families. Both his past experience and his Christian commitment, therefore, disposed him to be an engaged, discerning patient-customer. For his negotiating efforts, Roger achieved a discount of over 40% off the original bill total, leaving him with around $45,000 in remaining charges to be shared within the charitable network. The need was met.

Although this brief story ends well, it should give us a sense of how just a few trips to the hospital for anyone not loaded with cash could saddle an uninsured person or family with a serious depletion of capital, if not a mountain of fresh debt. It should also remind us that, however much we might try to prepare ourselves, we are not always ready for the curveballs Providence throws our way.

On that note, let me share a second story.

CLAUDIA'S STORY

Little Claudia Swanson was full of surprises from the start. The Hebrew meaning of her name, which her parents Jeff and Kelle chose before she showed up, is "lame" or "limping." But she was hardly slow to arrive once Kelle's labor pains began. In fact, she nearly made her debut before the midwife got there, no doubt giving mom and dad a newfound appreciation for the seasoned experts.

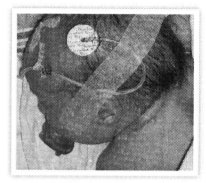

Claudia Swanson was born with Spina Bifida and was rushed to the hospital soon after her birth.

Claudia certainly stands out in her own way, wearing leg braces and requiring a walker to get around, but she is manifestly a Swanson. She finds herself surrounded by loving siblings. Her parents are people seasoned with a due sense of God's grace and wisdom even in his ordaining of difficult or challenging circumstances for his people. Jeff has a large, lumberjack build. To just look at him, you wouldn't necessarily peg him as a pastor. But he's kind of a gentle giant, deliberate and careful with his words and movements. Kelle struck me as a thoughtful person, attentive wife, and caring mother.

Soon after delivery, the midwife identified a smudge on Claudia's back which, when washed with saline, revealed an opening in her spine about the size of a Kennedy half-dollar. Spina bifida, they were told. The Swansons soon found themselves trailing an ambulance on a two-hour drive to a hospital in Grand Rapids, Michigan.

(We are not so accustomed to hearing about spina bifida sufferers today. The ability to detect fetal abnormalities together with our penchant for aborting "trouble makers" has seen to that. We've swapped trusting God for playing God.)

The primary health concern with spina bifida early on is that the back is open and the spinal fluid, which leads to the brain, runs the risk of being exposed to bacteria. This can lead to nervous tissue damage and infection. Spina bifida is also often correlated with a condition known as hydrocephalus, in which an abnormally high amount of cerebrospinal fluid accumulates in the brain, causing the head to expand and often creating various mental disorders. Thus, an initial key step in addressing Claudia's condition was to seal up the area at the base of the spine and closely monitor her during her first several days on the outside. Kelle recalls how quickly a rather routine in-home water birth led to an anxious trip:

> I had obviously just given birth, so my body was still recuperating. Within a half an hour maybe of her being born I was being put in a car and following her to a hospital. We took her to one hospital first and then they sent an ambulance up from a nearby children's hospital that had a little more specialized equipment… I think I was in shock to some degree at that point still, you know, not expecting that that was how things were gonna go!

Again, thankfully, like the Stubers, the Swansons were able to enjoy the fruits of heroic medicine and Claudia received the help she needed. But for all that, her start in life was certainly not without trouble. In her first month of life, Claudia had four surgeries. These included an immediate neuro-surgery to close the wound at the base of her spine, plastic surgery to separate her skin layers and replace them over the location of the wound, a repair surgery to re-close the wound after a spinal fluid leak was discovered, and surgery to shunt spinal fluid from where it eventually began to pool in her brain to the peritoneal cavity. All of this was, hands down, a tremendous blessing, thanks to modern science and industry.

But if you're not yet expecting to pay top dollar for the blessings of American health-care, expect to. For Claudia's care over just a two year period, the charges racked up to over $200,000 and her parents got to experience the sticker shock that is daily visited upon uninsured health-care consumers. Absent a pricey insurance policy and a pristine prior bill of health, a surgery ticket even within the ballpark of a quarter million would be enough to break most of us. To be sure, the Swansons found themselves roughed up a bit by the school of hard knocks that is medical billing in America and by the sheer largeness of the charges that accompanied Claudia's treatment. They were, for example, struck by what they found to be an "obscene" charge of $18,266.56 for a single MRI. Yet, however stunned, they were not threatened or undone by the weight of their financial obligations.

Their source of confidence amidst these challenges resided in a thoughtful Christian faith and a steadfast reliance on the mutual support found within the community of believers. Like the Stubers, the Swansons manifest this confidence and reliance through their participation in a specifically Christian health-care sharing organization. To the surprise of some of their friends and family members (and even, to some extent, themselves), the deliberate, voluntary giving of Christians enabled Claudia's parents to finance her operations and further treatment without being bankrupted. But that wasn't before they'd had a front row seat to health-care price inflation.

Questions arise, however, that are worth asking. What stands behind and accounts for the exaggerated costs so often bestowed as a sort of devilish parting gift upon cash-paying patients? Are there some greater social and economic realities that might help us to grasp why anecdotes like those shared above appear so common these days? How can we act to cure whatever it is that seems to be ailing the inflationary environment that is our health-care system?

BRILL'S "BITTER PILL"

Journalist Steven Brill takes a bold stance in identifying what he believes is the main dysfunction in U.S. healthcare:

> The issue of why the prices of health-care are so high is actually more important than the question of "who pays?". Because when you get into a debate about "who pays," you're just sort of moving the ball around... You're not really solving the problem. The simple problem—it's highly complex—but it boils down to a simple problem in this country is that the price for everything associated with health-care is just way too high... in comparison to what any other country spends, often to produce better results than we produce in the United States. Everybody's just making too much money, except for the nurses and the doctors who are providing the care.

In a lengthy March 2013 article for *Time* magazine, Brill documents some of the key problematic symptoms of a troubled U.S. health-care.

We interviewed Mr. Brill in his office high up in a skyscraper over-looking New York City. He came across as a straight-talking guy, donning suspenders and a red tie. He's just what you would expect if you were going to meet someone who's sort of a big deal in a big city.

Taking a "follow the money" approach, Brill emphasizes, for example, how providers mark up prices on goods. He cites the box of gauze pads that goes for $88 a pop to a self-pay patient—versus the $14 bill for the same box that would be footed by Medicare, which by statute must only pay what it cost the provider plus a little for overhead.

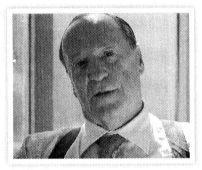

Moving toward a deeper diagnosis, he seeks to demonstrate that the health-care industry's providers of goods and services—in particular, the administrative executives of so-called non-profit hospitals—enjoy a "total leverage" over the buyers. In a move that fans of my last film *IndoctriNation*

Mr. Steven Brill, author of "Bitter Pill," talked to us about his research into medical billing.

will probably find more telling than he does, Brill suggests a comparison (only to fault it) between the sort of State-aided power wielded by teacher's unions—that has led to pricey but poor education—and the sort of financial wizardry and sleight of hand exercised by health-care plutocrats:

> My experience writing about education reform had told me that in that sector, which... is often delivered in kind of a monopoly way—the public education system—the teacher's unions had basically taken over the asylum and that's why education wasn't as effective in the United States and why it cost so much more than it does in every other country. So I thought, well maybe that's the case in healthcare too. And it turned out that those ideas were completely wrong and what was the real problem was that you had a marketplace that didn't function in any way as a marketplace. In any kind of real marketplace the buyer has some relevant balance of power over the seller. But in the healthcare marketplace the buyer has no power. The buyer doesn't know what the prices are and can't do anything about the prices even if he knows what the prices are.

It strikes me that Brill gets some things right and some things definitely wrong in his assessment. I think what's right about what he says has to do with the fact that a large segment of health-care consumers find themselves woefully deprived of information about prices—information that would prevent economic exchanges in this realm from one-sidedly benefitting one party (say, corporate executives) at the expense of another (say, patients or doctors).

Without going into how Brill overplays his hand in the extreme way in which he slights the effectiveness of American medicine (in contrast with the rest of the world), I think he's off-target when he presents things as if health-care price inflation is the result of some act of "capitalistic fiat" on the part of suppliers. As easy as it is to present things in a way that scorns "the rich," the inequities we witness today in health-care markets are not to be abstracted or removed from a complicated history in which the interface and exchange between doctors and patients has gradually suffered the growing involvement of various "interloping" third parties. We'll have more to say about this later.

Moreover, even my anecdote about Roger Stuber's ability to negotiate a lower price on his brain surgery shows that the soaring costs of care are not unilaterally dictated in the way Brill suggests. An engaged health-care consumer is a patient who is counting costs. He is one who economizes. As such, he acts in a more economical way than one who simply receives benefits on someone else's dime. He applies downward pressure on the costs of services by carefully limiting his consumption and by acting as a discerning shopper before he decides to buy.

What's further intriguing is that Brill raises the specter of monopoly in his comparison of health-care and the tight grip that the unions maintain within public education. P.J. O'Rourke, the satirist who coined the ironical phrase "wait until it's free" in reference to the looming costs of socialized health-care, has written about monopoly. In his book *Eat the Rich: A Treatise on Economics*, he writes:

> Any good drug dealer can tell you to ensure a monopoly, you need force. To ensure a large monopoly, you need the kind of force only a government usually has. And it still doesn't work.[3]

---

3   P.J. O'Rourke, *Eat the Rich: A Treatise On Economics* (New York: Atlantic Monthly Press, 1998), 111.

O'Rourke then goes on to discuss how the government of Cuba decided that beef cost too much and imposed sub-market prices on it. When that happened, the beef supply dried up and people were driven to create a black market in beef in which they paid the older prices. My point in bringing up the issue of monopoly is that if we see some market participants controlling prices as if to presume that consumers will not find equal or better options elsewhere, then we should be suspicious that a coercive agency—a government—has somehow helped to create an unlevel playing field (e.g., for health-care providers). I say this, of course, knowing some of the history of health-care in the United States, a history littered with government people committed to tinkering with and manipulating the marketplace (and a few too many non-government people okay with letting them do it). Could it be that this history somehow accounts for the marginalization of patients and doctors that Brill rightly bemoans? I think so.

And that's what this book is largely about. In working toward a more precise diagnosis of this problem, however, it will benefit the reader to gain familiarity with some of the history of Washington's attempts to involve itself in the world of health-care. In my judgment, it's not a pretty picture.

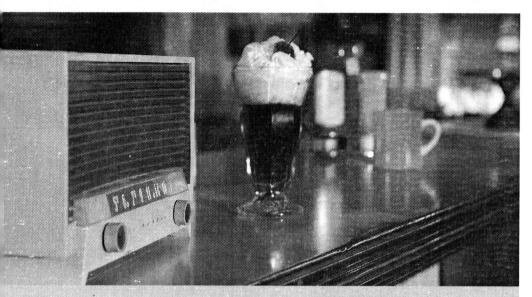

2 THE DESCENT (INTO HEALTH-CARE STATISM)

OUT OF THE HEART ARE LIFE'S ISSUES

"Keep your heart with all vigilance, for from it flow the springs of life."

The above passage comes from Proverbs 4:23 and draws an important connection between man's mental and emotional life and man's bodily life. On one hand, man is not a discombobulated gathering of electro-chemical events. On the other hand, nor is he essentially an immaterial soul trapped in a prison of flesh. Rather, he is a body-soul created in the image of God and

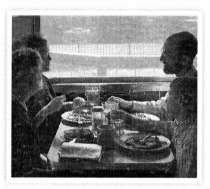

We look at some of the events that led to the change in affordability and the amount of government involvement in the health-care system.

designed for worship and service with his entire mental and physical being. Biblically speaking, the heart figures as the nerve center of man's thinking and actions. It's his base of operations. And the same goes for groups of people (i.e., societies). As they think in their hearts, so are they in life.

Sadly, the twentieth century witnessed some profound heart failures and these have had some negative consequences for the way human bodies are treated and cared for (or not) in the U.S. Along these lines, I want to begin here by drawing attention to a role that education played early in the twentieth century in helping to accustom Americans to an expanded role for the State in medical matters and correspondingly lesser institutional roles for individuals, families, and churches.

We look at some of the events that led to the change in affordability and the amount of government involvement in the healthcare system.

THE ANCIENT ART OF PHYSICIAN RATIONING

I'll start with the American Medical Association (or AMA) and how its organizers, via legislation and regulation, succeeded in placing downward pressure on the supply of physicians and a corresponding upward pressure on the price of a physician's services.

The AMA has played a pivotal role in promoting the professionalization of the practice of medicine in the U.S. Now, most of us will hear the word 'professional' and wonder what possible objections someone could have to such a thing. But it should first be understood that the professionalization that has come about due to the AMA's actions is not something that developed from "grass roots" or from tremendous market demand for stricter guidelines, expectations, or educational standards. Rather, it occurred in line with a vision and plan that some doctors had for imposing uniformity, at least partly for the purpose of restricting the number of those practicing medicine so that the incomes of those meeting "professional" standards would rise.[1]

Regardless, however, of the motives behind it, the spearheading of standardization took place in very much a top-down manner. The late Canadian scholar, Ronald Hamowy, states that the issue of education was considered to be so important by the AMA that at its founding in 1847

> one of its first acts was the establishment of a Committee
> on Medical Education which was to remain in existence for
> fifty-seven years, until replaced in 1904 by the Council on

---

1   Ronald Hamowy, "The Early Development of Medical Licensing Laws in the United States, 1875-1900," *Journal of Libertarian Studies* 3 (Winter 1979), 75.

> Medical Education, with greatly expanded powers to investigate
> and recommend improvements in medical training.[2]

By 1870, however, it was evident that the AMA was not going to have success in imposing uniform standards without the aid of legislative force. Realizing this already in 1867, the AMA members met in Cincinnati and endorsed a resolution urging their fellow doctors

> in the different States to use all their influence in securing such
> immediate and positive legislation as will require all persons,
> whether graduates or not, desiring to practice medicine, to be
> examined by a State Board of Medical Examiners, in order to
> become licensed for that purpose.[3]

While we today are conditioned to accept such regulative overreach as the norm—constitutional or not—in the nineteenth century it represented a significant interruption of free market forces. And I would contend that it did violence to the liberty of individuals to engage in relatively unencumbered exchanges with one another.

A generation later the AMA's success in wielding legislation and manipulating public opinion, in many respects for the benefit of its own members, was achieving new levels. As mentioned, in 1904 the Committee on Medical Education gave way to the expanded powers of the AMA's new Council on Medical Education. Four years later, in the interest of forming new standards by which to judge those operating within the medical marketplace, the Council asked the Carnegie Foundation for the Advancement of Teaching to survey American medical education. The result of the Carnegie study was the Flexner Report.

The Report did not disappoint the Council. Crafted by Abraham Flexner, it called for a reduced number of medical schools as well as physicians in the country. Toward that end, Flexner recommended that proprietary medical schools be shut down, that all medical schools be associated with a university, that stricter requirements be met in order to enter medical school, that medical school should comprise a more exhaustive schedule of study and training, and that there should be increases in state regulation of medical licensure.

2   Ibid., 75-76.

3   Ibid., 77.

The Report proved socially, legislatively, and economically important, exercising influence on the Federation of State Medical Boards, a non-profit organization founded in 1912 that, to this day, acts as a gatekeeper for those who would practice medicine.[4] As a result of Flexner, many medical schools shut down or were forced to merge with others, driving up the cost for those schools still in existence (illustrating the old law of supply and demand—when supply declines relative to demand, the price per unit of supply will rise). Naturally then the inflated educational costs were passed on from the physicians to their patients. But not all patients were able to absorb the new prices, so the provision of state-approved medical attention became, even more than before, the possession of wealthier Americans. This has, more or less, remained the way of things right up into the present. According to an AAMC study released in October 2013, the average new MD emerges from med school with over $150,000 in school debt.

No doubt, the restrictive standards of uniformity proposed by the Flexner Report and imposed by its heirs has helped to buoy the costs of health-care.

ROOSEVELTIAN REFORMS: ENCOURAGING DEPENDENCY AND INVITING THIRD PARTIES

So the expansion of State power didn't erupt from nowhere when FDR took office in 1933. There were precedents. All the same, only a fool would say that Roosevelt's presidency did not make strides in the direction of State-managed health-care.

First, under Roosevelt ~~the most successful Ponzi scheme to date~~ Social Security made its official debut. Social Security did not, in its original form, end up figuring prominently in the halls of socialized medicine but that was not for a lack of trying on the part of its designers. Originally, Social Security included a provision for a nationalized health service. As it became clear, however, that such a stipulation would kill the bill's chances, the bulk of the health service provisions were left out. Yet it is still the case that the signing of the Social Security Act of 1935 constituted a shift in what Americans stood for. We had become more secularized in that we were now comfortable with transferring the responsibility of providing a safety net

---

4   See Reuben Kessel, "Price Discrimination in Medicine," *Journal of Law and Economics* 1 (Oct. 1958), 20-53.

for the elderly and infirm from the personal touch of families and churches to a less personal and less capable centralized, redistributive bureaucracy.

After the advent of Social Security, there came stumbling upon the war-path the Stabilization Act of 1942. This lawless piece of law was apparently not a deliberate attempt to pave the way for an embrace of health-care collectivism. But in a blundering sort of way it had that effect. The Stabilization Act was Roosevelt's bumbling effort to suppress the inflation of American wages, comparable to the cartoon character who has two lumps on his head and so pushes one of them down only to have the other swell up propor-tionately. The Act prevented wages and salaries from being increased beyond the levels they were at as of

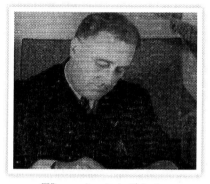

FDR was not content with having passed the Social Security Act of 1935. During WWII, he signed the Stabilization Act, a bill that prevented employers from raising wages.

September 15, 1942. Excluded, however, from these price controls were "insurance and pension benefits in a reasonable amount to be determined by the President."[5]

What resulted was the era of employer-sponsored health insurance in which we still find ourselves. This legislative artifact of FDR's amounted to a gargantuan subsidy and shot in the arm for those marketing pre-paid medical insurance. These latter were the supply side beneficiaries of the choices made by employers to attract employees by offering impressive, tax-deductible health benefits packages. In addition, Roosevelt's price controls gave patients financial incentives for signing over many of the economic decision-making duties related to their consumption of health-care goods and services to various third party payers. Thus, wittingly or not, FDR played a crucial part in converting patients from consumers into mere recipients of services. And when consumers cease engaging in careful cost-benefit analysis—when patients are separated from the payment for care—they will pay a high price for doing so, not only in how little control they have over the care they receive but also in the large number of dollars they must fork over for it.

---

5   Stabilization Act of 1942, § 10.

THE ADVENT OF MEDICAID AND MEDICARE

During the next two decades there ensued a growing debate over whether or in what way the Social Security system would be supplemented with a federal assistance program designed to procure basic medical care for at least some (presumably impoverished) portion of the population. The history of the legislative efforts and public discussion surrounding these matters is complicated. As an illustration, consider that the AMA consistently supported what was known as the Kerr-Mills legislation, which later, after some negotiated modifications, became Medicaid. At the same time, the AMA took a hard line in the late fifties and early sixties against the King-Anderson bill, which was an earlier incarnation of the substance that would later be named Medicare. Some of this history appears in Code Blue: Health Care In Crisis, a book by Dr. Edward Annis, the former president of the AMA responsible for rebutting President Kennedy's proposal to move America toward socialized medicine:

> Medicaid, as originally conceived (it has changed considerably), provided a cart for those who could not provide for themselves, but it did not burden the workers pulling the cart with unnecessary riders. The AMA fought the creation of Medicare precisely because it put everybody over a certain age in the cart regardless of ability to pay. In our objection, we correctly predicted the economic dislocations that currently plague the system, and noted that the dislocations would lead to a call by the political Left and the liberal media for more of the same; i.e., a completely socialist medical system.[6]

While I find reason to fault his earlier representative endorsement of Medicaid, Annis reasoned soundly with respect to some of the faults and fruits of Medicare.

In 1961, an actor named Ronald Reagan made a record titled "Ronald Reagan Speaks Out Against Socialized Medicine." There he articulated a commitment to free enterprise and exhorted his listeners to write to their congressman, making it known that they did not want governments

---

6   Edward R. Annis, *Code Blue: Health Care in Crisis* (Washington D.C.: Regnery Gateway, 1993), 102-103.

controlling businesses and industries. Referring to the King-Anderson (which later became Medicare) bill, he warned:

> If you don't [write your congressman], this [Medicare] program, I promise you, will pass just as surely as the sun will come up tomorrow. And behind it will come other federal programs that will invade every area of freedom as we have known it in this country. Until one day...we will awake to find that we have socialism. And if you don't do this and I don't do it, one of these days you and I are going to spend our sunset years telling our children and our children's children what it once was like in America, when men were free."

Since that recording was made, America has witnessed a gradual unfolding and fulfillment of Reagan's reluctant prophesies. It appears we have failed to heed well enough his warnings.

A few short years after an ambivalent Kennedy was out of the picture but before Armstrong had landed on the moon, the U.S. took one giant step in the direction of universal health coverage. In 1965,

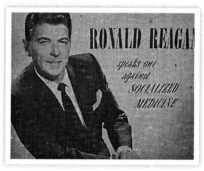

By 1961, the organizers of Operation Coffee Cup were opposing the encroachment of government into the world of medicine.

President Johnson signed the Social Security Amendments of 1965, thereby adding Medicaid and Medicare to the existing Social Security Act. Medicaid would combine federal and state funding to provide health insurance for those lacking the income and resources to pay for it. Medicare would force individuals to forego a consistent percentage of earned income in their working years, in order to number them among those who would receive old-age medical benefits once they reached the age of 65. Both programs signaled an amplification of State-dependency and Medicare especially acclimated Americans to coercive collectivism, encouraging them to have a sense of entitlement by first taking from them to pay for the elderly as a general class. Medicare also, it turns out, softened up Americans for a more all-encompassing welfarism that would take hold in the decades to follow.

THE GROWTH OF HEALTH-CARE WELFARISM UNDER THE CLINTONS

As we shall see, the expansion of the welfare state did not really take a hiatus over the next twenty-five years. Nevertheless, the Clinton regime that came to power in 1992 played a critical role in advancing America further down the road toward a single-payer health-care system. Yes, don't forget those Clintons. They helped to entrench us more deeply in the perverted ways of redistributive ninnyism.

Things got underway with the fight to get the Health Security Act (AKA Hillarycare) passed in 1993. Thankfully the bill ran into some powerful opposition and was defeated but not before floating some symbolically dense test balloons before the American public. The Clinton plan to socialize health-care from top to bottom included mandates that all citizens and permanent residents in the U.S. be enrolled in a qualified health-care plan and that employers furnish coverage for all of their employees. These details, I trust, ought to distinguish the Clintons' ideological efforts with a ring of familiarity in the ears of us beneficiaries/victims of similar recent legislative contrivances.

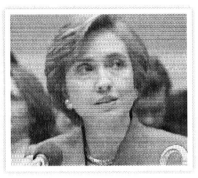

Even with multiple levels of federal and local health programs already in place, there persisted a desire to involve Washington in the health-care business. In 1993, the Clintons pushed for the passage of the Health Security Act, also known as Hillarycare.

After that main event got cancelled, President Clinton reached into his bag of collectivistic tricks for more. In 1996, he signed HIPAA, the Health Insurance Portability and Accountability Act. This was a dastardly document that plunged the government into all kinds of regulating and restricting of various group health-care plans and individual insurance plans. Also named the Kennedy-Kassebaum Act, after its two leading sponsors, HIPAA was designed to protect, through federal oversight, the health insurance coverage of workers who change or lose their jobs. Metaphorically, the law pours cement around the feet of the employer-based coverage that constitutes a significant portion of the American health-care system.

HIPAA has two key facets. Under Title 1, the Act imposes limits on restrictions that group benefit plans are allowed to place on benefits for pre-existing conditions. And this is just one part of the added red tape under Title 1. More generally, its mandates tinker with and in various ways undermine the ability of insurers to measure and manage risk by their own lights. Under Title 2, the Act stipulates that the Department of Health and Human Services (HHS) should create standards for the use and dissemination of health care information. While these changes help to cultivate the sort of information exchanges meshing well with a centralized, mechanistic system, the HIPAA requirements are so detailed and complex and come with such strict civil penalties for violation that attempts to comply with them have led to an entire industry of hired technocrats:

> How to correctly interpret and comply with HIPAA regulations has created a vast industry of consultants and technical advisors who have profited from the fears of physicians, medical institutions, and medically related companies and healthcare insurers.[7]

Giving a sense of the capital being diverted from arguably more productive uses, Dr. Peter Kilbridge in 2003 cited data from Healthcare Information and Management Systems Society and Phoenix Health Systems estimating the costs of HIPAA "to be...more than $1 million in 16% of large hospitals (i.e., in those with more than 400 beds)."[8]

Having long since distanced himself from the path of wisdom, Clinton in 1997 launched SCHIP, the State Children's Health Insurance Program. With the bipartisan sponsorship of the ubiquitous Teddy Kennedy and Utah's Orrin Hatch, under SCHIP the federal government provides matching funds to states, procuring insurance coverage for families with children. In particular, SCHIP brings into the fold of the State's dependents children in families whose incomes are low but not quite low enough to qualify them for Medicaid benefits. At its creation, SCHIP figured as the largest expansion of taxpayer-funded health-care provision since LBJ signed his approval of Medicaid in 1965.

---

7   Deeb Salem, "HIPAA's Privacy Regulations: Increased Privacy Comes at a Cost" at http://www.medscape.com/viewarticle/461703_4; Internet; 2 August 2014.

8   Cited in Salem, "Regulations," 2014.

REPUBLICANS IN A SUPPORTIVE (EVEN INNOVATIVE) ROLE

It's important also to acknowledge the contributions of those Republicans who helped to bridge the way from LBJ to Bill Clinton's programmatic ramping up of health-care statism.

For example, as if to remove any doubts about his questionable economic judgment (after he had imposed Rooseveltian price controls and ended convertibility of the dollar to gold on a single day in September 1971), Richard Nixon signed the Social Security Amendments of 1972. By doing so he welcomed to Washington's dole those who have been severely disabled for over two years and those who have end stage renal failure disease. And this sort of misguided Republican compassion didn't end with Watergate.

Even with his reputation for fiscal conservatism, Ronald Reagan did things that encouraged health-care providers both toward a dependence on State funding and also toward economic waste. In his second term, he signed EMTALA, the Emergency Medical Treatment and Active Labor Act (1986). The act requires hospitals that accept Medicare payments—those that are equipped to evaluate and treat outpatients for emergency medical conditions (which is almost all hospitals)—to "provide emergency health care treatment to anyone needing it regardless of citizenship, legal status, or ability to pay."

On the positive side, patients without any sort of insurance or welfare coverage are still reckoned under the law as legally responsible for the costs incurred for any such care. On the negative side, EMTALA keeps so-called private hospitals fastened to the teat of Medicare by mandating that they dole out the services. As if that was not enough, outlays for these "free" services are not directly covered by the federal government (one of those notorious "unfunded mandates"). No wonder, then, that the Centers for Medicare and Medicaid Services reported in 2007 that 55% of emergency care goes uncompensated.[9] The results of this have consisted of cost shifting (which has meant inflated bills for those who can pay) and some rather coercive "charitable" write-offs. Sadly, this was a major motion toward universal health-care thanks to one who had earlier crusaded against it.

---

9 "The Uninsured: Access to Medical Care," http://web.archive.org/web/20090116041157/http://www.acep.org/patients.aspx?id=25932; Internet; 11 October 2014.

In 1989, Reagan's motion got a hearty second from an unexpected section of the "conservative" choir, The Heritage Foundation. It may come as an unspeakable shock to devout Republicans but President Obama appears to be a Johnny-come-lately at the Individual Mandate party. That's right, the individual mandate has a sweet Republican history. It was unabashedly put forward as a solution by Stuart M. Butler, PhD, in a 1989 "Heritage Lectures" publication titled "Assuring Affordable Health Care for All Americans." As the second of several "key components" deemed necessary to reform health care (for example, dealing with the middle class "free rider" problem), the author stipulates: "Mandate all households to obtain adequate insurance." Butler himself, I learned, has been an outspoken realist about the budgetary crisis surrounding Medicaid, Medicare, and Social Security. However, due to his willingness to mandate the purchase of health insurance (or any type of insurance!), his credentials (and those of Heritage more generally) as a true mouthpiece for economic liberty have been sadly tarnished. This is especially the case for anyone willing to see the resemblance between his recommendation and the offerings of Obamacare.

Not enough embarrassing facts? How's this one? A piece of legislation in 1993, introduced by Senator John Chafee, set a further precedent by taking Dr. Butler's advice. The Health Equity and Access Reform Today Act coupled a requirement to have health insurance, with a penalty for non-compliance, with government-subsidized, state-based "purchasing groups." The Repubs, you see, were serving up a mix of "death to liberty" and crony capitalism that the Democrats have only recently mastered. Want to know something else? There was a notable silence from the Republican ranks in the teeth of this mischief. In general, Republicans did not do much hollering about the constitutionality of such a proposed law, not to mention it being an offense against private property and true free markets. How could they? It turns out, after all, that a crucial facet of Obamacare was copied and pasted straight from an old Republican playbook. The playbook came from the likes of Mark Pauly, who had helped develop a proposal similar to Chafee's for President George H.W. Bush. That was the era of Bush the Elder.

Then came Bush the Younger's turn. President George W. Bush, I want to believe, was a well-intentioned man. But he never struck me as one who was brimming with careful thoughts about how economies work and how governments are generally a hindrance to economic flourishing.

As evidence of this, even before he went on to "save capitalism" by agreeing to have taxpayers bail out failed banks in the 2009 financial crisis, Bush approved the largest expansion of Medicare since its inception in 1965. This came in the form of the 2003 Medicare Prescription Drug, Improvement and Modernization Act. The Act, which took effect in 2006, ushered in what was known as Part D, a prescription drug benefit. Also called the Medicare Modernization Act (MMA), Bush's law has multiple complex facets, which cannot all be explored or even summarized here. Suffice it to say, Medicare Part D blends Bush's unquestioning promotion of the economic insanity that is Medicare with the government's subsidizing of large insurers and HMOs. This built upon Nixon's initial fascistic favoring of HMOs (which we will touch on in a later chapter) while setting a further precedent for Obamacare's recent protection of larger insurers and networks through its health insurance exchanges.

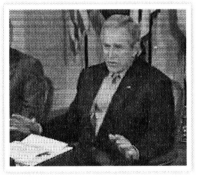

In 2006, Republican President George W. Bush passed legislation subsidizing the purchase of pharmaceuticals for the elderly.

One sad fact is that older Republican readers of this book are much less prone than their parents or grandparents to sympathize with the judgment of the previous paragraph—that Medicare embodies economic insanity. When one spends one's entire adult life having a portion of his wages systematically, involuntarily transferred to elderly beneficiaries, it's easy to gravitate toward a "now it's my turn" mindset. The presence of such a mindset helps to account for how Republican politicians have become what they used to criticize (i.e., demagogues, vote-sellers). It's the same mindset that accounts for "Hands off my Medicare!" signs turning up at Republican conventions.

It is true that in a couple bouts of good judgment inconsistent with his own expansion of Medicare, George W. Bush rightly vetoed two attempts to expand Clinton's SCHIP program. Rather astutely, he argued that these were federalizing moves that would "steer the program away from its core purpose of providing insurance for poor children and toward covering children from middle-class families." On these occasions, Bush well enough grasped that the SCHIP program promised to transform members of the "host" (the taxpayers) into parasites (tax beneficiaries). But that bit of good sense was just a little water in the desert, especially given Bush's failure to uphold such principle on a consistent basis. And his successor has only dug deeper into the wallets of taxpayers and victims of Central Bank inflation.

Last but not least, we would be remiss if we didn't mention Romney-Care. It's no secret that former Governor Mitt Romney's health care reform law of 2006 served as a prominent model for the Obama administration's Affordable Care Act. Let's not forget also that this was a law generally approved and passed by a *Republican* governor. So the Fox News warriors and other *Republicanistas* who dump exclusively on Dems the blame for our woes should give the two-party hobby horse a rest. Having caught the sick proclivity (from those like Heritage and the Clintons) for creating market demands by legislative dictate, Romney signed his approval of a general mandate that Massachusetts residents purchase insurance, extended "free" health insurance for residents earning less than 150% of the federal poverty level, and required employers with more than 10 full-time employees to provide health-care insurance.[10] Translation: the Republicans do not have clean hands.

Moreover, it is not at all clear that RomneyCare brought healing to Massachussetts. For instance, in a 2010 interview, Romney was confronted with the fact that emergency room costs had increased 17% in the last two years.[11] In the same interview, he was unable to explain exactly what problem RomneyCare solved. Of course, this might be understandable if we'll consider that Massachussetts had the highest per capita health-care costs before RomneyCare and since.[12]

Along with this unhelpful attack on private property at the consumer end of things, Romney also did the K Street dance. Specifically, he conspired to funnel mandate-induced business toward certain chosen insurers. He did this by establishing the Commonwealth Health Insurance Connector

---

10   Thankfully, the employer mandate was repealed in 2013. See Matt Dunning (2013), "Mass. Health care reform law's employer mandate repealed," http://www.businessinsurance.com/article/20130717/NEWS03/130719866/mass-health-care-reform-laws-employer-mandate-repealed; Business Insurance; Internet; 16 October 2014.

11   See Dale Steinrich, "100 Years of US Medical Fascism," http://archive.lewrockwell.com/steinreich/steinreich12.1.html; Internet; 30 October 2014.

12   See "Health Care Expenditures per Capita by State of Residence," http://kff.org/other/state-indicator/health-spending-per-capita/; The Henry J. Kaiser Foundation; Internet; 30 October 2014.

Authority (CHICA). Serving as a microcosm of Obamacare's insurance exchanges, the CHICA plays the part of a broker, directing residents to "approved" insurance plans.

These earlier Republican precedents thus supplied more recent players on the other side of the aisle—such as Kathleen Sebelius, Nancy Pelosi, Harry Reid, and Barack Obama—with some important political building blocks with which to build.

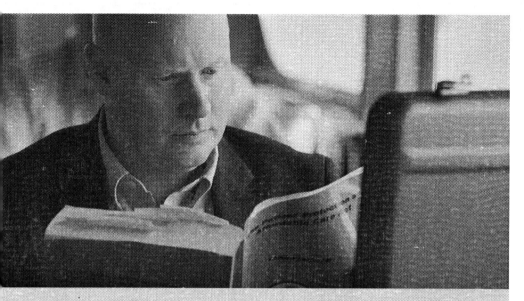

3 DOUBLING DOWN ON A BAD IDEA: "OBAMACARE"

On February 4, 2009 the still freshly elected President Barack Obama signed the Children's Health Insurance Reauthorization Act of 2009. Standing on Clinton's pandering shoulders, he looked to advance the perception of D.C. as America's chief breadwinner and provider of hospitality. It would be hard to say he failed to accomplish that, no? He successfully arranged for SCHIP to include an additional 4 million children and pregnant women. President Obama's expansion of the SCHIP program was, of course, just a drum-roll. It was an indicator of and prelude to something much larger and more fearsome that was soon to make its way down the pike.

We may look back and remember the Affordable Care Act ("Obamacare") for the vapid one-liners associated with its arrival and the underhanded way it came to be law. In March 2010, House Speaker Nancy Pelosi insulted the intelligence of Americans with the phrase, "We have to pass the bill so that you can, uh, find out what is in it." A little later, in 2014, a series of videos surfaced featuring an MIT economics professor, Jonathan Gruber. In the videos, Gruber can be heard citing "the stupidity of the American voter" as a justification for the deliberately "tortured way" in which the ACA law was written in order to obscure the centralizing, socializing aims of its architects.

Although, if we look back in ten or twenty years and mostly remember the silly and duplicitous ornaments adorning Obamacare's arrival, that's probably a good sign. Perhaps that would mean that the substance of the ACA had been scrapped a while back for something less bad (let's hope), with little remaining but the sadly entertaining quotes attending its advent. I say this partly because I'm inclined to think that if Obamacare is the wave of the actual future, then it is more likely that we'll hearken back as those who look through a dark, dense fog, barely able to recollect the good ol' days.

The fog would consist of the social and economic results of the current doubling down on the religion of Statist Intervention. Because of the amplifying of coercive wealth redistribution and marketplace manipulation, we face the prospect of stifled competition, higher costs, less care, and less quality care. To sum up, we should be realists and expect a drop in our health-care standards. Unfortunately, it's not the easiest thing to show that a certain policy (the application of a politico-economic philosophy) has had negative economic consequences.[1] Something I'm keen to focus on, however, is the fact that our economic outlook as Christians is rooted in a more all-encompassing spiritual and moral worldview.

Along with many Christians and other liberty-minded people, I oppose those who would seek to consolidate power and authority within the realm of the secularized State. Those with an understanding of that thing called Christendom will understand that individuals are sovereign, families are sovereign, churches are sovereign, and civil magistrates are sovereign. Even apart from that, each individual bears the divine image and therefore owes fidelity and obedience to the Creator over and above any honor given to Caesar. But in defending this viewpoint we also ought to seek a clear understanding of our intellectual and political opponents.

Along these lines, one does not have to be a very astute observer to recognize that Barack Obama, Kathleen Sabelius, Nancy Pelosi, Harry Reid, and the like are true believers in Big Government. If they were to stamp their ideals on a coin, it would read "In the State's competence to Unite and Provide we trust." Andrew Schlafly, General Counsel for the Association of American Physicians and Surgeons, sketches in broad strokes the mindset of these people and their liberal forebears:

---

1 For a text that explains how significant social and economic damage can be done by government interventions without being easily noticed, see a recently republished version of Henry Hazlitt, *Economics in One Lesson* (Auburn, Alabama: Ludwig von Mises Institute, 2008).

The Left in America has been trying for fifty years to get control of the health-care system. And that's for a variety of reasons. One is it's a big portion of our economy. It's one-sixth of our economy. So if the government can exert control over such a big chunk of our economy, then the government's expanded its power and it's exerting the type of command-and-control system that the Left wants to do. That enables the government to dole out benefits as they do in Canada. When it gets close to election time in Canada, all of a sudden care is given out more freely. And then the voters are more *appreciative* of the incumbents in power and they tend to vote for the incumbents.

This reflects the politicized, demagogic perspective on the world that the current president and his political allies share. Schlafly is one who should know something about this, having served side-by-side with the "aloof" Obama on the Harvard Law Review during their days in law school together from 1988 to 1991. It was evident to Schlafly even then that Obama was "not a friend of free enterprise," a quality that has persisted into the president's middle age.

However, even though Obama blends a propensity for exercising coercive controls over medicine with precious little *medical* knowledge, he has done some learning about

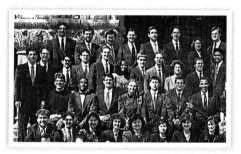

Andrew Schlafly (second row from the top, second from the left) and Barack Obama (second row from the bottom, on the far right) worked together on the prestigious Harvard Law Review.

politics in his life. In particular, he's done well enough to see that reaching the goal of a single-payer health-care system is like eating an apple: it is best done one bite at a time. More specifically, he grasps that even with our incremental drift toward interventionism and centralization over the past century the empowering of the State in the United States is most effectively done by *capturing* and *compromising* American businesses. This approach allows the "hosts" (agents of economic productivity) to go on living and earning, while allowing political demagogues to manipulate markets and further their reputations as the politico-economic saviors of the parasitic *hoi polloi* (which, oddly, includes the likes of both favored corporations and impoverished welfare recipients).

If you are following the trail of bread crumbs I'm leaving, you can get a sense of how President Obama got the tragic ACA law passed. With some skill, he mixed together a commitment to *secular collectivism*, a willingness to embrace *crony capitalism*, and a talent for *community organizing*.

When you think about it, the Affordable Care Act is a uniquely American piece of socialistic legislation. On the one hand, Obama and his like-minded colleagues and political allies have, for years, desired to exercise social control in a way that would bring about guaranteed health coverage for all Americans. (We won't here explore the many possible deeper motives for this.) On the other hand, they have also faced (ala Hillarycare's defeat) the political reality that a single-payer system following the models of Canada or Britain is still a pretty tough sell in the States.

So, there's the *what*—government managed health-care—and the *how*—the recognition that this should take the form of pretending to operate still within the context of market forces and competitive corporate interests. The ACA appears to offer just such a magical elixir, but magic can be a messy business. It sometimes blows up in your face, and it's usually not what it appears to be but is rather a bit of skillful sleight-of-hand.

The chapters that follow will go deeper into my understanding of the problems of our health-care arrangements in America and their solutions. First, however, it deserves mention that, although the liberals may be off-target in their own proposed solutions (and without reservation I assert that they are), they perceive correctly that something is broken in U.S. health-care. It's nevertheless my contention that they go wrong in diagnosing the exact nature of the problems and therefore proceed to offer solutions that are themselves problematic. They end up throwing good money after bad (or at least bad money after worse money) and succeed in *lowering* our standard of living. Enough caveats though.

With the announced goal of expanding both public and private insurance coverage and also reducing costs in both domains, Obamacare attempts to overhaul American health-care by dictate. The tools of the trade include mandates, subsidies, and exchanges. To add to this general characterization, allow me briefly to summarize and comment on three specific pillars that make up "Obamacare": the employer mandate, the individual mandate, and the State-subsidized insurance exchanges.

THE EMPLOYER MANDATE

To begin with, the ACA lays down an *employer mandate*. This is an aspect of the law that may have shocked even Roosevelt's sensibilities. The employer mandate requires people who have 50 or more employees to offer those they hire on a full-time basis a health insurance benefit. Failure to comply with this requirement has consequences in the form of tax penalties.

The employer mandate made its way into the ACA, first of all, due to the prolonged attachment of Americans to employer-provided insurance coverage. This is something we discussed in an earlier chapter. A 2013 Kaiser Family Foundation study, for example, showed that, of the 80% of Americans with health-care insurance, 54% have coverage furnished by their employer.[2] The designers of Obamacare did not appear practically interested in questioning the overall benefits of employer-based coverage.

One who wishes to insert between doctors and patients an additional, vast apparatus of bureaucrats and third parties, after all, is not prone to placing the focus of his critique of the present system on the encroachment of third parties into the doctor-patient relationship.

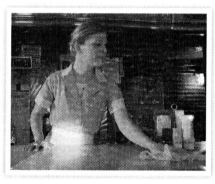

On the other hand, integral to the ACA is the way it brazenly imposes standards for what constitutes acceptable insurance plans, the way it privileges certain select insurance providers, and the way

By forcing the link between employment and health insurance, one intensifies the problem of "job lock," in which employees remain wedded to their jobs in order to maintain health insurance coverage.

it threatens to (and does) steal money ("funds") from those who forego insurance. We have apparently drifted far enough down the road toward the Secular State that we now know about "the Exchanges," in reference to the coverage dealers commended to us by the Washington Overlords. But the

---

2   "Health Coverage & Uninsured," http://kff.org/state-category/health-coverage-uninsured/; Kaiser Family Foundation (June 20, 2013); Internet; 29 October 2014.

"system" forged in the fires of the ACA is a patchwork system. It takes what was already there and tacks on a bunch of other junk. That's where the employer mandate comes in. It's part of the junk.

There is some advantage for the social engineers in D.C. to have "qualifying," employer-based insurance plans remain in place for many people. The ACA's attempts to maintain and upgrade plans offered by employers can be thought of as one manifestation of the political reality that the American people seem not quite ready for the sorts of disruptions they would be treated to if the liberals got their way and inflicted upon us a single-payer health-care system like one finds in Canada or Europe. In view of this political reality, the current health-care "markets" must remain in place (like a flimsy veneer), while numerous new impositions and penalties are used to effectively *socialize* health-care costs. As one part of this, business operators must be forced to buy more insurance for their employees or else suffer the wrath of the IRS.

These are the attitudes and political realities that proponents of health-care liberty must confront. Looming larger, however, is that dreaded product of Neo-Con creativity in the late 1980s: the individual mandate.

THE INDIVIDUAL MANDATE

Back in 1994, in the teeth of both Republican and Democrat efforts to use coercive means to have Americans acquire health-care coverage, the Congressional Budget Office (CBO) issued a report describing an individual mandate as

> an unprecedented form of federal action… The government has
> never required people to buy any good or service as a condition
> of lawful residence in the United States.[3]

This, I must say, is not altogether true. Individuals are threatened with and often go to prison should they decide against "volunteering" tax returns or payments to the IRS.[4] The tax payments are then used to pay for various

---

3   Quoted in Katharine Q. Seelye, "Court challenge seen in health insurance mandate," *New York Times* (Sept. 27, 2009); http://www.sfgate.com/news/article/Court-challenge-seen-in-health-in-surance-mandate-3216886.php; Internet; 1 November 2014.

4   Filing a tax return is "voluntary" because otherwise the IRS, by requiring a person to file a tax return, would violate an individual's 5th Amendment right to not witness against himself. Want to win $50,000? See if you can meet William Conklin's challenge: http://www.givemeliberty.org/people/billconklin.htm.

goods and services. Nevertheless, even agents representing the CBO twenty years ago felt that an individual mandate figured as a fundamental threat to property rights.

What is the individual mandate?

The individual mandate sits at the heart of the ACA law. Unlike even the employer mandate, it is an *essential* part of the Obamacare "engine." The mandate requires that all individuals not sponsored by an employer, Medicare, Medicaid, or other such financial assistance provider (or better, *appropriator-distributor*) purchase an "approved" private policy or pay an annual tax penalty.[5]

So there are real costs incurred for socializing costs, aren't there?

To use a line from Jean-Jacques Rousseau, we were born free(er) but are everywhere in chains.

The importance of the individual mandate for Obamacare can hardly be exaggerated. It's really a matter of funding. If certain privileged insurance providers are to grant everyone some semblance of coverage, then they must be in a position to finance the costs incurred. Many of those previously viewed as greater insurance risks, for example, due to preexisting conditions, must now be brought aboard the insurance bus. The insurers, along with the administrators of Medicare and Medicaid, are the drivers of the bus. Understandably, bus drivers who are forced to cram in more noisy passengers want to be paid for their trouble.

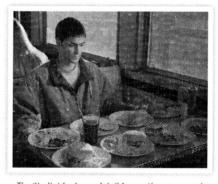

Meanwhile (sticking with the bus analogy), some of those who have been riding the bus for years

The "individual mandate" forces the young and fit to buy insurance that they don't want or need.

are going to get less attention and service from the bus driver. Also, the bus driver's fees stand to increase, as the lowered standards necessary to

---

5   We will see in Chapter 11 that amidst the many tyrannical details of the ACA law there resides an exemption for those belonging to a qualifying health-care sharing organization. Members of such an organization are loosed from the requirement to prepay for health coverage or pay a tax penalty.

include all riders will marginalize competitive transportation services. What the individual mandate does is require people to board the generic, yellow bus (as there are fewer competitors among insurers due to cronyism). Because some of those aboard the bus cannot afford the driver's fee (not to mention the fees of the bus manufacturer and bus mechanic), others will face either higher costs (in the form of premiums or deductibles, leaving aside taxes and inflation) or further rationing of their own care by subsidized insurers. One of the morals of this story is that an acquisition of *formal coverage* should not to be equated with an acquisition of *material care*.

Here we've touched on things from the angle of the consumers of coverage. The individual mandate permits our central planners to *broaden the risk pool*. But what about how things look from the angle of the suppliers? What about the insurers?

STATE SUBSIDIZED INSURANCE EXCHANGES

If someone's buying, someone's selling.

If there's to be a chicken in every pot, someone must dispense the chickens (no matter how pesky or riddled with steroids the chickens may be). Imagine the "insurance exchanges" as a taxpayer-sponsored farmer's market. The market is open only from October 15th to December 7th each year. But don't get too excited. Not everyone is allowed to deal his wares. We wouldn't want the customers to have too many options! Most anyone should have access to most any product at a reasonable price (i.e., a price the taxpayers can afford to pay).

To put it bluntly, the ACA law is where genuine health insurance—rooted in actuarial tables and proper risk assessment—went to die. Under ACA's provisions, something called *guaranteed issue* prohibits insurers from curtailing or denying coverage in view of a person's pre-existing conditions. Walking hand-in-hand with this silly stricture is the requirement that insurers offer all applicants of the same age and geographical region the same premium price—or *community rating*—irrespective of pre-existing conditions.

Add to these repudiations of fiscal prudence and economic liberty the fact that Uncle Sam is subsidizing certain providers and insurers who are able and willing to adapt to the mandates, comply with HIPAA, etc. Is that what government is supposed to be about? No. Doesn't this amount to playing favorites and manipulating markets? Yes. But since when did that stop us? Nixon was sponsoring HMOs 40 years ago.

Also factor in an amendment of the ACA, the Health Care and Education Reconciliation Act (HCERA), signed on March 30, 2010, which requires health plans to provide "first dollar" coverage for certain preventive services free from cost sharing requirements. What this means is that the insurer is on the hook from the start, with no co-payment or deductible levied on the insured as an out-of-pocket cost for the services received. Such economic silliness reinforces the already dysfunctional habit we Americans have of converting an instrument best used as an emergency backstop (in the case of a catastrophe)—health insurance—into a way to pre-pay for our consumption of certain goods and services. When placed before the public as a taxpayer funded provision—entrusted to managers with no skin invested in the game—this sounds like an excellent way to encourage overconsumption, create shortages, and generate reactionary attempts to ration care according to the priorities of a collection of bureaucrats.

All of this awaits us in sizable doses! Though I hope not really.

Anyway, in the next chapter, I will go further into a subject (which I've just mentioned above) relating to the unholy marriage of government and corporate interests. For short, we can call it corporatism or crony capitalism. From what I hear, it's pretty standard fare in a place called K Street.

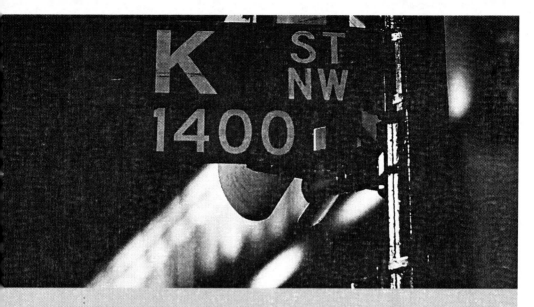

4   K STREET SHENANIGANS

In the face of their own finitude and the reality of economic scarcity, people aspiring to god-like status tend to resent their shortcomings and seek "work arounds." Historically, this is a tendency among tyrants and government execs. When, for example, Moses and Aaron approached the Pharaoh, requesting that Israel be released to hold a feast to the LORD in the wilderness, he said, "Who is the LORD, that I should obey his voice and let Israel go? I do not know the LORD, and moreover, I will not let Israel go." After that, he commanded taskmasters of the people:

> You shall no longer give the people straw to make bricks, as in the past; let them go and gather straw for themselves. But the number of bricks that they made in the past you shall impose on them, you shall by no means reduce it, for they are idle. Therefore they cry, 'Let us go and offer sacrifice to our God.' Let heavier work be laid on the men that they may labor at it and pay no regard to lying words.[1]

Pharaoh was an economic planner who wanted more for less, maybe even something for nothing. He was unwilling to reduce his output demands

---

1   Exodus 5:7-9

in light of a curtailed supply of integral inputs. There are still people who think that way.

Before we get to that, however, let's ask ourselves: all other things being equal, would it be better for all people, regardless of income or social standing, to have affordable access to the highest quality healthcare available? I wager that, for the most part, fans of bigger and smaller government alike would answer this in the affirmative. I agree that it would be better.

But the Stubers and Swansons and Steven Brills of the world are onto the fact that something is askew in health-care. The prices tend to be intimidatingly, often bankruptingly high. There are hospital chargemaster rates, for example, old prices—still on the books—that have no rhyme or reason to them and yet to which cash pay patients are exposed. Unlike insurance outfits or corporate giants, uncovered individuals are not in the anointed position that would typically allow for the type of fat discounts that can be achieved on a massive group plan.

The uninsured are like tiny, hungry goldfish in a large lake with a moderate supply of food. They have also been growing in numbers. This means more goldfish and likely *more gaunt* goldfish.

Not surprisingly, health insurance premium costs have proved a more faithful indicator of the Federal Reserve's unrepentant cheap credit policies over the past two decades than have income averages. As a partial result, it's become increasingly sensible for individuals to opt out of the health insurance market. This fact also goes along with an American insistence on using insurance to finance day-to-day medical expenses, a relying upon third parties for counting costs and rationing consumption, and the ongoing unemployment associated with stock bubbles and bank bailouts.

So, what's the solution? From a formal economic standpoint, there are three possible answers to the high prices and/or diminished supply of something: 1) increase the supply of the desired goods and services, 2) decrease the demand for those same goods and services, or 3) accomplish some combination of both.

On one hand, of course, governments are not really good at creating things. Okay, foreign scandals and domestic messes, maybe. (For an illustration of the latter, think of the embarrassing rollout of the Obamacare exchanges.) Enough said. On the other hand, there are still people like President Barack

Obama, who are committed to chasing the fox of universal health-care with the understanding that the hunt is best undertaken with the bloodhounds of taxation, regulation, and redistribution at one's side. To use another metaphor, when they went about their health-care reform efforts those of Obama's politburo and its congressional allies were not interested in making or baking a whole new cake. Appropriately. In engineering Obamacare, they were all about forcefully re-slicing pieces of an already existing cake. As government employees, they were limited to manipulating forces on both the side of supply and of demand to at least give the impression that the State is the preeminent Provider of health-care.

Like a bloodhound himself, Tim Carney, Senior Political Columnist at the Washington Examiner, has a nose for Washingtonian naughtiness. He has skillfully reported on how the Affordable Care Act became law and why it took the shape that it did. In particular, Carney has addressed questions concerning why the Democrats and Neo-Cons have yet to furnish us with a single-payer system as we see elsewhere in the Western world and how corporations and powerful industries managed to figure so prominently in Obama's reform package. Recall, after all, that while he was on the campaign trail Obama marketed himself as not only a friend of the poor and working class but also as an opponent of special interests, such as corporate lobbyists. But his presidential self, according to Carney, has not cracked up to be what his candidating self led folks to expect.

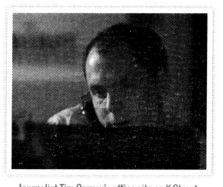

Journalist Tim Carney's office sits on K Street. He has earned a reputation for carefully researched journalism about how lobbyists have come to have a shaping influence on legislation as well as market forces.

Arriving with our crew in Washington, I hoped that Carney would help us in exposing some of the latest in political pragmatism. We met up in a spacious newsroom late at night with our lights, cameras, and questions ready. If you ask me, it felt a little like we were shooting a scene out of *All the President's Men*. We were there to blow the lids off a few secrets. Thankfully, our source didn't disappoint:

President Obama did come into office promising to battle the special interests but he certainly didn't. (And even if you look at his campaign finance money, the drug industry and even the insurance industry gave more money to him than to John McCain in the 2008 election. In fact from the drug industry, he brought in record amounts of money.) But then, when he came into office, he did work hand in hand with the biggest lobbies.

This reveals hypocrisy and expediency, yes. But it also reveals an entire lobbying industry that rewards and is itself rewarded by those in positions of political power:

> If you want to understand Washington, I always say, you have to understand Congress and the White House, but the other important branch is what we call K Street. It's a street here in town, but it's sort of the proverbial corridor of lobbying. So, you have lots of lobbying firms that represent a number of companies. You have lots of industry groups representing, say, the drug industry or the oil industry or the hospital industry. And all of these lobbying groups hire up former congressmen... former congressional staff. And then those lobbyists have tremendous influence, in part because they're raising money for the congressmen, in part because they're calling their old friends, their old colleagues, their old bosses, and they're saying, "Here, you need to listen to my views on this policy." And that's one of the most powerful forces in shaping policy here in Washington.

MEET THE CRONIES

When the enormity and influence of the various groups related to American medicine and health-care are taken into account, it is little wonder that these companies and sub-industries have molded legislators and legislation. Carney rattled through some of the culprits:

- "The single biggest lobbying entity that represents a single industry in Washington is the Pharmaceutical Researchers and Manufacturers of America. It's a drug lobby; they abbreviate it PhRMA. They spend more than any other single industry group in all of Washington. And if you were to take the... industry as a whole, counting the drug companies that they represent, then that is the single biggest industry. You may think that the oil lobby or big tobacco spend a lot. None of them spend nearly as much as the drug industry."

- "The American Medical Association is the biggest lobby representing doctors and the American Hospital Association represents the hospitals. Both of those lobbies ended up supporting Obamacare pretty firmly. And I think both of those industries profit from it."

- "The health-care industry has a smaller industry called America's Health Insurance Plan. AHIP, as they call it, made sort of the opening bid in Obamacare after Obama was elected, where they said they would cover everybody, everybody's pre-existing conditions, as long as everyone was forced to buy private health insurance."

Touching the third bullet point here, imagine guaranteeing Americans a "chicken in every pot" by forcing everyone to buy a chicken! Resorting to such measures was not originally in line with Obama's *modus operandi*, but he was a practical enough man that he eventually caved to the hard line taken by one such as Hillary Clinton.

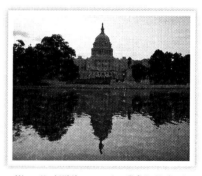

But this is not your grandfather's garden-variety socialism. The individual mandate achieves a double whammy. It makes citizens further beholden to their overlords. True enough. On top of that, however, it offers protection—by way of statute— to those insurers willing to bow to an

We waited till the sun set on D.C. to find out how deals are really made in Washington.

imposed set of minimum standards for health insurance policies. Although, as Carney notes, the insurance lobby appears to have benefited the least in contrast to other health industry lobby groups, it's still not too bad a deal to have civil penalties out there "encouraging" people to consider your products. Never mind that some shoppers seeking low premium, high deductible plans may be ushered toward the very opposite. To take things in a more clownish direction, why should nuns be stuck with contraception coverage? And why should any man be insured for lactation consultations?

The absurdities could be multiplied, like clowns piling out of a car.

Such corporate pandering may not strike everyone (like it does me) as an offense against liberty and property. But at least consider that there are actual negative economic consequences for those who would otherwise compete with those companies capable of hiring the attorneys, accountants, and lobbyists to smooth the way toward their enrichment. Also consider the consequences for consumers who now will have both the fewer options and higher costs that result from a "fixed" market:

> The drug industry got a few favors that could end up costing you too. For example, the [ACA] bill includes *twelve-year monopolies* for the big biotech companies on their biotech drugs. That means that cheaper generics don't get to come on until twelve years after the biotech drug goes on. With regular drugs it's five years. So, if you *have to buy* the name brand drug, this means that some medication is going to cost you *much more*. And Obamacare was the law that created the twelve-year monopoly on biotech drugs.

> Again, the drug industry, especially the ones that make these high tech, biotech drugs, was a firm supporter of this bill, was raising money for democrats who would support it, and they ended up winning, while consumers end up losing.

Other wounds dealt to the free market include the subsidies paid to drug companies for the purpose of expanding Medicare Part D's prescription drug coverage. Lucky (rich) stiffs.

TWO KINDS OF ENTREPRENEUR

So who's responsible for helping to limit consumer choices and restrict competition, nay, for working evil against the recipients and would-be providers of innovative, diversified options for medical care? To mention two: a smattering of State Agents and their Corporate Allies, no doubt. And let's not pretend to be surprised by this. K Street was, after all, busy with traffic long before "Big Pharma and the Insurance Giants" were out there on the corner banging out the hits.

The practice of cozying up to a coddling congressman in order to gain subsidies and stymie one's rivals dates back at least to the nineteenth century. A great place to start reading about this is Hillsdale historian Burt Fulsom's book *The Myth of the Robber Barons*, where he distinguishes between market entrepreneurs and political entrepreneurs.

Market entrepreneurs, on one hand, have been those who slave to offer goods and services that consumers will favor. Failure for them amounts to the inadequate provision of things and actions that are pleasing to consumers. Profit and loss is what it's all about. Political entrepreneurs, on the other hand, are those who—perhaps weary of creating, innovating, and serving—have turned to buttering up the powers on high in hopes of getting some legislative Kryptonite in return, a bit of magic from the gods of Washington that will cripple competitors, or at least keep them at bay. Far too often, they've been met by elected officials and entrenched bureaucrats who are all too willing to play ball. But the boys and girls of D.C. and their corporate bedmates can't run the sneak play around straight dealing and basic economics forever without somebody noticing.

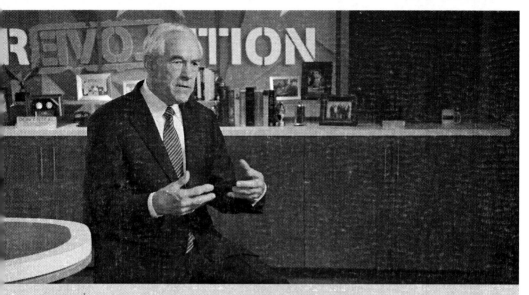

5 DR. RON PAUL TAKES ON DIM-WITTED DO-GOODISM

AN AGENT OF RESISTANCE

In December of 2013, by a gracious providence, I had the privilege of meeting and interviewing someone who most certainly has noticed the shenanigans over the years and has not stayed quiet about it either.

After two months of patient but eager anticipation, our crew set out for Clute, Texas, a city just south of Houston on the lower east side of the state. Among other things, Clute is famous for a fossilized mammoth that was once discovered there, which is probably fitting, since the man we were on our way to see spent much of his professional career squaring off against a living, breathing mammoth that lives near the Potomac River—the beast of D.C. politics.

From what I've been able to tell, the former Texas congressman's interactions with Washington for the past four decades have had less to do with *impressing* someone in order to gain further tenure and more to do with *impressing upon* his colleagues, constituents, and anyone else who would listen what he believed was the right and prudent thing to do for his constituents, his country, and the human race. I believe this helps quite a bit to explain his significant popularity among young, independent voters. He's taken on the role of a fatherly teacher, who's well acquainted with the foolhardy attempts of governments and bureaucrats to intervene in and manage people's lives.

I'm afraid, however, that many who may have been exposed to Dr. Paul through mainstream media sound-bytes—for instance, the presidential debates—might tend to perceive and remember him as a reactionary figure.

That would be a schoolboy error. Not only did his actions as a legislator from very early on center around a studiously considered understanding of government under the U.S. Constitution as being limited to several enumerated powers, he has also shown himself to be a lucid proponent of free markets from the standpoint of economic analysis. Indeed, his principled approach in these areas came across clearly in my interview with him about the state of American health-care.

IDENTIFYING THE PROBLEM

Like a physician forming judgments about a patient's condition, we should not be content to dwell on the symptoms of our country's faltering health-care arrangements without seeking to diagnose their underlying cause(s). For example, consider as a disturbing symptom the increasing costs in medical care and as another a growing number of unfulfilled doctors and alienated patients. Do we face these realities due to a lack of government programs or interventions into the medical marketplace? Dr. Paul doesn't think so.

For starters, along the lines of what we discussed in an earlier chapter, he acknowledges that the past half-century witnessed various state efforts to control and manage the world of medicine:

> Like so many things in life and society, governments incre-
> mentally invade... the people's rights and privileges... From the
> beginning, it was just one program after another... Medicare
> and Medicaid came in after I had my medical degree... But it's
> gradually increased over the years... those programs, they've
> expanded... and I always thought it was a bad sign, going in the
> wrong direction.

Those who are pushing for universal care on the order of Canada or France should thus be honest with themselves. Or, if that's asking too much, they should ease up in their demonizing of free markets and admit that a good bit of welfarism, regulation, and market manipulation on the part of the feds predates the winter of our present discontent. So, let's disabuse ourselves (and those we meet) of the idea that a free market in health-care has been recently tried and found wanting. Rather, it's been incrementally left *untried.*

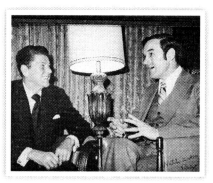

But the question still stands. From whence cometh the escalating costs one incurs for being wheeled down the all too lonely and bureaucratic halls of American health-care? For his part, Dr. Paul traces our malaise to a degenerated

Pictured here are two of the most politically influential and beloved "Ronalds" of the past 50 years.

doctor-patient relationship and places no small part of the blame on persistent government tinkering. He has consistently viewed government interventions as not safeguarding but rather undermining the doctor-patient relationship:

> My biggest gripe about [government's involvement in the health-care business] was a medical gripe... It bothered me that it was going to cause a disruption of the doctor-patient relationship. And it certainly has... Today you can recognize how difficult it is to identify with a single practitioner.

Even with the best of motives, he contends, legislators and executives of the past century have had a hand in loosening patient-physician ties.

DOPEY, CONCEITED ECONOMICS

There are those who intellectually disagree. Some economists, for instance, account for the shriveling percentage of people able to afford health insurance premiums in terms of our heightened technological capabilities and a proliferation of potent pharmaceuticals. Now, certainly, we have a good deal to appreciate and be thankful for with respect to modern medical advances. The advent of infection-controlling agents (e.g., penicillin), laser technology, and microscopic surgical techniques has brought about a medicinal revolution resulting in longer life expectancy. Those children, for example, who survive the womb today only to get childhood leukemia, rarely die from it. In 1950 they rarely lived. And we pay for such benefits. We have paid.

But a net upward trend in health-care costs is not necessarily a result of higher quality. Indeed, accounting for inflation, we generally purchase better quality products today (cars and computers, to mention a couple) for less cost than we did fifty years ago. Dr. David Gratzer, author of *The Cure: How Capitalism Can Save American Health Care*, puts it this way: "A bulky calculator in 1972 cost 31 hours of work. Today, a more compact and more powerful one can be had for less time than a leisurely lunch: 46 minutes."[1] What then accounts for the fact that health-care costs have evidently not followed suit?

Let us come and reason together, making no mistake. The Affordable Care Act is a stride right in rhythm with a parade decades in the making. A little history can go a long way.

Strike one: since the late 19th century, states have, through licensing laws, imposed restrictions on the supply of doctors. Now, everyone knows that when the supply of a good is suppressed or limited, the price per unit increases. Thus patients are made the "captives" of an elite class of doctors, thanks to coercive restrictions (and if you think this is overly dramatic, try practicing medicine without a license). Licensing has, it stands to reason, resulted in less personal care, due to a disproportionate ratio of patients to doctors. In other words, through physician licensure, state governments have been busy *rationing* health-care provision for over a century.

Strike two: an elected leader called FDR imposed limits on the price of labor in 1943. As market actors adjusted to this intrusion, the era of employer-provided health coverage was born. Effectively, the federal government subsidized the rise and expansion of the third-party payer system we now know by imposing price controls and by making employer-provided health insurance tax-deductible. This pushed costs up by taking patients—those previously prone to act as consumers engaged in cost-benefit analysis—and transforming them into a more passive lot, shielded from the duty of calculating and rationing for themselves. Now, don't we all

---

1   David Gratzer, *The Cure: How Capitalism Can Save American Health Care* (New York: Encounter Books, 2006), 34.

know that when a consumer is desensitized to the immediate costs of something, he will be less restrained in his demands and desires, leading to supply shortages and higher premiums? Additionally, by arranging (on purpose or not) the "wedding" of would-be patients to their employers and various insurers, a paternalistic politician encouraged the presence of middlemen. This creates administrative layers that compete with patients for a doctor's loyalty while adding to the overall expense of care. Hence, Roosevelt's attempt to manage markets arguably moved us toward less personal care that costs more. Thanks, FDR.

Strike three: there came along in 1973 President Nixon and his sidekick, Senator Teddy "Chappaquiddick" Kennedy. Together they passed the HMO Act, requiring companies that offered health coverage to include a managed care product. They stuck their oversized noses into markets and succeeded in underwriting certain industry players at the expense of others. By requiring coverage-providing employers with a certain number of employees to purchase an HMO product, the planners chased away marginal competitors with HMOs and thus relieved the latter's administrators and practitioners from having to battle as much for "customer loyalty" through service to patients. End result: fewer options, stymied innovation, and higher premiums.

Against the backdrop of this narrative, Dr. Paul corrects those who associate the shady activities of corporate cartels (represented, for example, by drug industry lobbyists) in places like K Street with a *laissez faire* approach to markets:

> This has nothing to do with free markets, even though they're corporations... People think, 'oh, the problem we have today is all because we have too much freedom and too much free enterprise' and we have none. We have government and big business in collusion with each other to... actually... force the cost of medical care up. Profit is delivered to people other than the people who... deliver the benefits to the patient.

What we should desire instead is a safe environment in which parties can participate in mutual exchanges whereby both benefit:

> As bad as our society is today, consumers are pretty good!... They don't go out and buy a used car carelessly. They're pretty

good at finding out what the price is and what to pay. And they do that with computers and cell phones and everything else. And the relative freedom that we have in these other areas... guess what? We find out the price is going down... So, the market is just begging and pleading to help out and yet all we get from Washington is obstructionism. Alw ways getting in the way. Always the do-gooder that's going to save the world and make sure everybody has perfectly equal medical care... and they're going to make it cheap... and exactly the opposite occurs.

I agree with what he's getting at here. Competition generally leads to better quality and lower prices, a proposition iterated in a 2014 article by Willem Cornax, who writes:

The successes of the free market you see all around you are within anybody's reach as long as there is real competition and not a sanctioned obligatory purchase of a service, for which the supply is then shared between a few large companies.[2]

Sadly, Dr. Paul is also right that there are many genuinely well-meaning people who go in for the idea that we don't have enough government in our lives. They are do-gooders who go about meddling, supposedly leveling the playing field and making things right. But I also think that at the core of much of this sort of thinking there resides conceit—the presumption that technocrats are sufficiently competent and virtuous to determine what we need and who should pay for it.

And when we talk about health-care, we're obviously talking about something that has more profound implications than the answer to the question, "How much is this going to cost and who's gonna pay for it?" We're confronting very emotional and important issues. Because sometimes we do really need a particular kind of drug or surgical procedure and without it we may die. Rightly, therefore, Dr. Paul has made a point of opposing the politicization of the marketplace—not least of all, the medical marketplace. Do we, after all, think that patients and consumers are likely to gain the undivided loyalty and help of a politician who is in thrall to a

---

2   Willem G. Cornax "How Third-Party Payers Drive Up Medical Costs" at http://www.mises.org/daily/6891/How-ThirdParty-Payers-Drive-Up-Medical-Costs; Internet; 2 September 2014.

company that's set to profit whether or not a patient, say, gets enough of a particular variety of drug which, if it were available in generic form, would be cheaper and more readily accessible?

I don't see why we would.

Let's pray that the Lord sends us more Ron Pauls and fewer Ted Kennedys. Can I get an Amen?

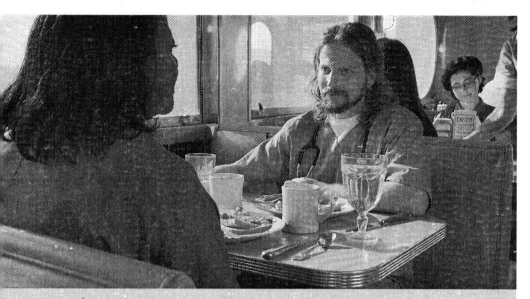

6 FIGHTING THE GOOD DOCTOR'S FIGHT

HEALING WHAT'S BEEN TORN

It may not seem initially obvious, but it's nonetheless true that two distinctive demons haunting health-care in America today are, one, a disengaged patient and, two, a distracted and thus disloyal (to the patient) doctor. By saying this I don't mean to malign physicians as a species. No more, anyway, than I'd want to put the slap-down on generations of patients who've grown up largely unaccustomed to thinking of themselves as discerning market participants in the health-care arena.

Okay, maybe I'm scolding a bit.

Taking a broader view, most of us find ourselves as pipsqueaks within a system that includes massive hospitals, insurers, networks, and conglomerates. These are the organizations that largely "own" doctors and thus—perhaps unwittingly (or perhaps not)—subordinate the once critical patient-doctor interface to various corporate and collective interests. Such colossal arrangements and institutions are the results of many layers of legislation, regulation, and social change. They didn't appear nor will they disappear overnight.

Recall, though, the words of a famous hobbit who said, "There's some good in this world, Mr. Frodo, and it's worth fighting for."

One thing that I do reckon to be good—some would even say sacred—and definitely worth fighting for is the relationship between a doctor and his or her patient. So, though I started this chapter by casting a qualified insult at doctors (and patients!), the remainder focuses on ways in which physicians have, along with their patients, been betrayed by third-party interference.

PROTECTING THE PATIENT'S INTERESTS

In important ways, the doctor-patient relationship survives today as a sort of conceptual relic. It's not very common, say, to have a single family doctor whom you inherited from your parents and pass on to your kids when you pass on, like you would precious metals. At one time in America, however, the family-doctor relationship was a treasured thing.

Again, don't get me wrong. By the Lord's kindness, we in the West especially have enjoyed the fruit of scientific and technological developments that permit us to live longer and more comfortably. But one can also become so enamored with the accoutrements and devices as to allow a personal and spiritual component to drop from view. So, I ask: have we been guilty of trusting supplemental technology, powerful narcotics, impressive buildings, and so on, in such a way as to stifle a more primal concern we would otherwise wish to promote, namely, the concern to heal the sick and promote health? There's a case to be made that we have. Yet I've become convinced that our failures in this area work to the detriment not only of patients but also of physicians.

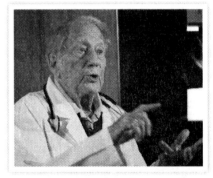

In this connection, I had the opportunity to interview and capture on film Dr. Curtis Caine, a man who has fought for decades to prevent third parties from playing anything more than second fiddle to the patient-doctor relationship. It was a delight to meet Dr. Caine.

Before retiring, Dr. Curtis Caine opposed the socialization of health-care throughout a lengthy and illustrious career in medicine.

Not only did he educate me about how the quality of doctoring declines when third parties play a lead role, but he also came across as a very genuine and generous person. I have to think that for his many loyal patients the experience of knowing him must have been quite similar.

By no means, however, has his stand for the primacy of the patient been restricted to the privacy of an office. In a very public way, Dr. Caine has actively and winsomely sought to resist the interposition of government regulations and rules between health-care providers and their bosses, the patients. A simple Google search of his name, for example, leads to a letter he wrote in the year 2000 (found on the website of Hacienda Publishing) in which he maintains that a proper understanding of Article I, Section 8 of the U.S. Constitution would forbid Congress from making laws regarding medicine.

He's written other letters as well, one being particularly noteworthy. In it, he recalls:

> Back in 1965, Medicare was proposed and instituted by the government to go into effect in a few months. In 1966, I wrote a letter and mailed it independently, mimeographed it myself, addressed it myself, stamped it myself to every one of the nineteen hundred doctors then practicing in Mississippi... In that letter, I presented the case against Medicare. I listed 122 reasons why my colleagues should turn down being participants in Medicare and begged them... to resist intrusion and to not get suckered into Medicare.

As is evident from his humble but thundering epistle, Dr. Caine understood that Medicare was far from the final chop into the tree of life, liberty, and free market medicine. The wielders of the axe intended their program as an opening move toward federally procured care for all Americans, not just the elderly. He also understood what sort of waste and mediocrity had taken up residence in the numerous countries that already, at that time, opted for socialized care. He was thus inclined to issue warnings and cite examples:

> The Italian Mariotti Project would nationalize all physicians. Canadian medicine is again the target of the socialist government. Mexican, Swedish, German, Czechoslovakian, Hungarian, Libyan, Cuban, Polish, Bulgarian, Rumanian [sic], and Chilean

medicine is socialized, and struggling with difficulties. Russian socialized medicine is experiencing shortages. Greek socialized medicine is, this month, plagued by exposure of corruption, fraud, and abuse.[1]

Sadly, this voice crying in the wilderness fell on too many deaf ears. In the ensuing months and years, flocks of physicians—those belonging to the class best positioned to put the kybosh on collectivistic care—did a kowtow and signed on to participate in Medicare.

So, doctors have, themselves, ceded much ground to the planners and interveners. They're not mere victims of third-party villains, any more than their patients are. We are, after all, citizens too. And too many citizens in the medical profession have gone along to get along, consented to the disrupters, and agreed to do their bidding.

Acknowledging this, I want to train our attention a bit more on Dr. Caine himself, as he doesn't exactly fit into this theatre of the absurd. If only we had more "sore thumbs" like him. In particular, I believe that his words as a faithful patient-advocate and his works as a tireless medical servant jointly testify against those—be they government employees or "health-care industrialists"—who allow patients to be displaced as the physician's chief professional loyalty:

> I had a love affair with medicine for sixty years. I characterize it as being selfless… I sweated, I cried, but I loved it. When I was putting forth my efforts, it was for the patient. Others were not involved. Third parties were not in my thinking… I didn't go into medicine to get rich. I did go into medicine to have a personal relationship with patients.

His devotion to his patients, moreover, stimulated a striving after excellence, an appreciation for the uniqueness of individual patients, and a propensity for creativity and innovation.[2]

---

1 Curtis Caine, "Dear Esteemed Colleague," at http://www.aapsonline.org/caine-letter-1966.pdf; Internet; 2 August 2014.

2 For a closer look at my interview with Dr. Caine and several other individuals featured in *Wait Till It's Free*, consider becoming a Backstage Pass Member. You can get started here: http://www.wtifree.com/coffeecup/.

To those who do get the chance to view the entirety of my interview with him, it should be evident that Dr. Caine views utopian social planning as a major source of mischief that has harmed the world of medicine. Yet, paternalistic Statism, while figuring prominently in his evaluation of our present condition, is not his only target. He identifies a more general threat, which he calls the interloper. An interloper is one who gets involved in a situation in which he has no proper place or business:

> If you understand a little organic chemistry, then you understand the difference between a straight chain three-carbon atom and a circular three-carbon atom... In the practice of private medicine, it's straight chain. You have the patient, who has a relationship with his doctor, and the patient, who has a relationship with a third party... The patient is the one who is the controller of the three... When you go to the... circular [holding up his fingers in the shape of a triangle]... then, the patient has a relationship with a doctor and the doctor has a relationship with the third party. And that dilutes... The relationship [between doctor and patient] is diluted, the responsibility is diluted.

I share Dr. Caine's concern that a dilution of the patient-doctor relationship in recent decades, being at least partially a result of doctor disloyalty, has worked to the detriment of patients. Indeed, the latter increa singly resemble a collective "third wheel" just grateful to tag along and be part of the excitement going on around them.

AAPS: OPPOSING STATIST INTERLOPERS

But let's not kid ourselves. Uncle Sam, the Interloper-in-Chief, has done more than his share to cultivate dysfunctional relationships in the medical community. To this the members of AAPS—the Association of American Physicians and Surgeons (AAPS)—can surely attest. For seventy years, AAPS members have battled Washington's attempts to shift market participation and responsibility away from patients (consumers) and physicians (voluntarily paid servants) to tax-funded regulators and various corporate cartels. With Drs. Paul (a member) and Caine (a past president), AAPS doctors have acted as brokers of liberty and private property, believing that consumer-serving markets best allow for the flow of information to and from providers. This not only tends to reduce costs but also improves the delivery of goods and services.

In 1943, AAPS took shape as a collection of doctors from all 48 states came together to oppose the Wagner-Murray-Dingel bill. The bill, which would have added health insurance measures to the already existing Social Security Act, went down in defeat despite the support it got from the National Farmers Union and several other organizations. The newly formed AAPS—which went on to adopt the motto *omnia pro aegroto* (Latin for "all for the patient")—together with other groups such as the Insurance Economics Society of America and the Pharmaceutical Manufacturers' Association, succeeded in killing the bill in committee. It fell like a castle, crumbling into the swamp that is Washington.

In 1993, exactly fifty years after being founded and with much water under the bridge, AAPS had occasion again to defy the Centralizers. As the virtual keystone in the arch of his first term, President Clinton unveiled a plan to provide universal healthcare for Americans. It was known as the Health Security Act. Within its more than 1,000 pages, the plan included as its central feature a federally enforced mandate for employers to provide health insurance coverage for all of their employees. Again, AAPS stepped up against what the Heritage Foundation described at the time as a "command-and-control system of global budgets and premium caps, a superintending National Health Board and a vast system of gov-

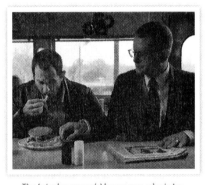

The Interloper could be anyone who interferes with the actions of a doctor or the choices of the patient. It could be a government agent or any other meddlesome third party that tries to interrupt or control the doctor-patient relationship.

ernment sponsored regional alliances, along with a panoply of advisory boards, panels, and councils, interlaced with the expanded operations of the agencies of Department of Health and Human services and the Department of Labor, issuing innumerable rules, regulations, guidelines, and standards."[3] It too fell into the swamp and died in Congress.

---

3   Robert Moffit, "A Guide to the Clinton Health Plan," at http://www.heritage.org/Research/Reports/1993/11/A-Guide-to-the-Clinton-Health-Plan; Internet; 2 August 2014.

Then, in the spring of 2010, a castle was erected through chicanery of all sorts. And it stayed up. For now.

ACA: EQUALITY SOWN, MEDIOCRITY REAPED

How does the Affordable Care Act offend liberty and sneer at good economics? Let me count the ways. By prohibiting insurers from denying individuals coverage due to pre-existing conditions (and other such measures), ACA charges at the insurer's right to transact freely while spearing sound actuarial practices of risk assessment. By reflecting the disregard of its architects for balanced budgets (and their swooning admiration for money printers), ACA feeds a parasitic mentality in its expansion of Medicaid eligibility to include households with incomes up to 133% (at least) of the federal poverty level. But for a moment let's ignore these unignorable details.

Let's focus instead on that *individual mandate*, the requirement that those not covered by their employer, Medicare, or Medicaid must either purchase a federally subsidized insurance plan or pay a tax (AKA penalty). Let's not think about how it infringes on the right to forego the purchase of a product (or about how a similar individual mandate appeared in a bill proposed by a Republican Senator in 1993). Instead, I want the reader to consider the individual mandate as an act of economic manipulation. I'm especially concerned with how it will impact the supply, the quality, and, if you will, the philosophical temperament of physicians.

Essentially, the individual mandate (along, it's true, with other parts of the ACA, such as the expansion of Medicaid, whose help comes from Central Bankers) procures and expands market share for its approved insurance dealers by securing an IRS-enforced financial incentive for folks to sign on with them. It's about creating jobs, you see. By legislative fiat, Obamacare generates a ready *supply* of federally approved "insurance" providers to meet the *demand* encouraged by the tax threat. There's a strong tendency to want to get something for one's own money, after all, if not for someone else's money.

What will be the impact of this mandate? I'm thinking in the direction of the doctors. Well, for one, it will place an upward pressure on the number of patients clamoring for care. Like the prodigal son making his way to the Statist swine trough, who isn't tempted to want dad to provide the goodies now, rather than inherit a savings plus interest later? When you're covered, you take advantage of it. No harm done to your wallet, at least not immediately. But then, what if everybody's doing it? More bids, higher bids, rising costs. And what is it buying?

It is conceivable that the government's efforts to guarantee customers will create incentives to enter the medical profession for those happy to eat scraps from a federally subsidized table. But physicians whose accounts are padded by persons other than their patients will reckon themselves *accountable* to those administrative networks and government rules. He who pays the piper calls the tune. We can thus prepare for a further indus-trialization and depersonalization of healthcare, an arrangement in which doctors-on-the-dole take to tuning out the needs and desires of their patients.

If you doubt it, see how things are working out for the British.

But there are also plenty of marginal players who have been cut off at the pass in their efforts to practice medicine, thanks to Washington's imposition of new

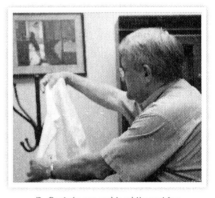

Dr. Beaty hangs up his white coat for the last time, on the day of his retirement.

and expanded administrative layers and compliance demands. In the film, we met Dr. William Beaty. He was the MD in Waco who, after facing the prohibitive costs of converting patient files to an electronic medical records database, ended his practice as a surgeon despite a few more years of work otherwise left in him. What tipped the scales was the effective elimination of his practice from the local referral loop as hospitals in the area scrambled to place all primary caregivers under contract.

Here we witnessed the ouster of an otherwise competent and com-petitive surgeon's practice. This is really a story of disenfranchising and discouraging small, personal service for the sake of a centrally ordered, clockwork efficiency. Dr. Beaty was forced out largely due to circumstances beyond his control.

Of course, life sometimes goes that way. No pity parties here. But I was quite impacted by the burden that smaller medical practices, in particular, carry in their efforts to keep up with all the regulations concerning the storage of medical records on file, the transfer of paper to electronic files, the costs involved for these things, and the ways that the imposed administrative layers distract practitioners from tending to the health and well-being of their patients. I felt myself surrounded by masses of files and nearly tripping over boxes that line the floor, and that's without even cracking the door of the warehouse Dr. Beaty required for storing older records.

One moral of this story is that we need more, not fewer, doctors in this country. According to Peter Fine, president and chief executive officer of Banner Health in Phoenix, the shortage in doctors is not a "looming" problem but a present reality. Consider that one out of three practicing physicians in the U.S. are over the age of 55, a good portion of whom are expected to hang up the white coat over the next ten to fifteen years. This, together with other discouraging statistics, instills no confidence that Obamacare's expanded crowd of not-so-calculating consumers (not to mention our aging Baby Boomer population) will have their insurance dollars met with prompt physician care.

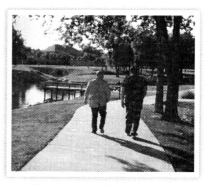

A walking interview with my friend Brandon, a medical intern who explained the massive sacrifice it takes to become a physician.

My friend Brandon, who by now has nearly completed his residency, is quite familiar with not only with the rigors of medical training but also the various stumbling stones confronting those on that route. Acquainted with Brandon through church, I found it impossible not to admire him as he strolled into worship a bit bleary-eyed and still in his scrubs. Feeling called to serve as a medical doctor even while married and with children, he gave up his chiropractic practice to plunge into the rigors of medical training.

As we saw in the film, medical students who are not independently wealthy are heavily leveraged when they emerge from med school. It's little wonder, then, that younger physicians are increasingly aspiring to specialized niches within the medical community. As a professor of medicine at the University of Washington (Seattle), David Dale says those seeking to specialize often do so as a result of cost-benefit analysis. Primary-care physicians generally work more, earn less, and face greater malpractice risks.

In considering the plight of those training to be full-fledged physicians, I recently struck upon an interesting comparison. If you talk to someone who works in the intelligence community, they'll confirm that spy agencies are especially careful to keep tabs on the financial condition (debt levels, etc.) of their employees and prospective employees. The reason for this is very simple. A person whose financial house is not well ordered or who is seriously cash-strapped will be more susceptible than otherwise to compromising his principles and loyalty. Once compromised, he will at least prove less effective in serving his employer's interests and may even work to the latter's disadvantage.

Although it's a dramatic example, I think this is the position in which we tend to place would-be physicians. Moreover, unless they are apt to cast off the preponderance of third parties, both corporate and governmental (between which the difference is ever shrinking), incoming physicians must readily acclimate to a principle of "the patient comes second (if she's lucky)." This falls short of an important ideal, one that the members of AAPS have upheld for 70 years.

The prospect of a company of doctors preoccupied with staying afloat financially or with pleasing parties other than those they're supposed to be caring for and curing is a scary one, but it's a matter of genuine concern. As a bankrupt Washington ratchets up the rationing of care in the coming decade, the planners and those who answer to them will visit upon us the sick underbelly of a collectivism that's coming home to roost. Death panels are no longer unimaginable. That's the way the UK has gone and the U.S. is never too far behind.

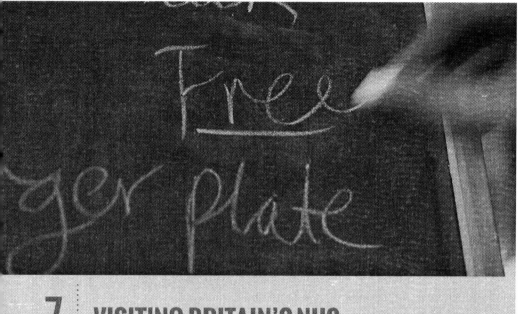

7 | VISITING BRITAIN'S NHS

SIGNS OF MORAL HAZARD

Returning home is always a pleasure. I live in Texas but most of my family and many of my friends live in Scotland. Going home usually means cooler weather and many meetings with close friends. But the Scotland I know doesn't exactly match up to the American imagination, which tends to drift quickly to thoughts of shortbread boxes, bagpipes, and William Wallace.

The romantic notion of Scottish life, however, is quickly quashed when you arrive in Glasgow. Not too far from the scenic Highlands (Scotland is a tiny country), Glasgow is a modern, formerly industrial, city. Hamilton, where I'm from, is only 20 minutes east, just a bit further up the Clyde (River). A great town, Glasgow nonetheless has its fair share of roughness, grime, and poverty—things common to the west of Scotland.

Health is also a big issue. Scotland is not so much *Braveheart* country as it is heart disease country. It's also fair to say that Scotland is suffering from a general health crisis. Much of it is tied to deviant behavior that is generations old. To cite an illustration, the county of Lanarkshire, where Hamilton is, contains an area known as the "Buckfast Triangle." Buckfast is a "tonic wine" (ironically brewed by some esteemed Benedictine monks) that is used in such profligate ways, mainly by young men, that, in the space of two recent years, the wine was mentioned in 6,500 police reports. An article on British news website DailyMail.com estimated that around $9 billion is spent overall by the NHS *each year* in dealing with medical problems related to alcohol abuse.[1]

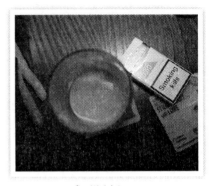

Scottish leisure:
Pints, pies and a packet of "fags."

Whatever should be further inferred from these facts, at the least they do not persuade me that nationalizing health-care services is the way of fiscal prudence, physical wellness, or moral uprightness.

In fact, a major complaint I have against making the State the manager of health and welfare relates to the *moral hazard* one tends to find within the enclaves of coercive collectivism. People who are consistently, institutionally prevented from feeling the economic impact of their decisions (through losses and rewards) will tend to take the ball and run with it (and I'm thinking of rugby here, not American football). Being relieved of the burden to care for their own selves and their dependents, they will too often accept that state of affairs and relinquish their sense of personal duty. Practically, this phenomenon manifests itself in a citizenry that feels entitled to certain State-procured benefits, the people's minds being dulled to the fact that economic resources are not infinite.

In our visit to Scotland, one of the friends I was able to go see was an old schoolmate, Pamela. She's a colorful character who recalled her experiences in the Scottish Ambulance Service. Specifically, she remarked about how emergency vehicles are frequently referred to as the "big white taxis," often being side-tracked into whisking the dissipated and indigent from the gutters and alleyways. In her time with the Service, she came across some of the "knock on" effects that accompany the collectivizing of costs. Namely, when people have the impression that a service is "free," their demand for that service is virtually boundless. Also, when your answer to the over-consumption of something is to continue furnishing an unabated,

---

1 "Alcohol abuse 'costing Britain £6 billion a year'," http://www.dailymail.co.uk/news/article-19699/Alcohol-abuse-costing-Britain-6bn-year.html; Internet; 6 January 2015.

taxpayer-funded supply of that thing, you get more of the wasteful, abusive behavior. Go figure.

In addition to underscoring these economic truisms, however, I want to say something here about one of Glasgow's famously besetting sins—drunkenness. Not only does a widespread idolization of booze by the city's inhabitants underscore the problem of overconsumption in the socialist commonwealth, it also should teach us that the effects of a particular health-care policy are not morally neutral. No doubt ambulances and ER wards have their place. But when the latter are consistently packed out like an Elton John concert and doctors are tempted to prescribe crowd-slimming placebos, it's time to indict a philos-ophy and government policies that effectively subsidize reckless living and the abuse of services.

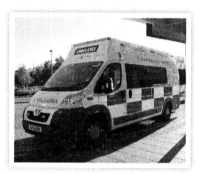

A "Big White Taxi" sits outside a hospital in Wishaw, Scotland.

Indeed, with the broadening of the State's taxpayer-supported shoulders in Scotland (or elsewhere in the UK), are the State's beneficiaries encour-aged to morally distinguish between a moderate, measured use of health-care services and an egoistic, cosmetic use of them? Not hardly. Under Britain's National Health Service (NHS), the patient menu today includes procedures such as breast enlargement, sex changes, in vitro fertilization, and abortion. This assortment of vanity and perversity is part of the mess of socialist pottage for which the UK, a while back, traded much of its productivity and dignity. It's a history that Americans would do well to heed.

THE NHS: ENVY OF THE WORLD (OR PERHAPS NOT)

The 1940s appeared a splendid time to push collectivist statism in the West. Like their Allies across the Atlantic, the British were pulling together to fight an enemy. It was thus in an era of togetherness and sacrifice that the National Health Service emerged.

If the NHS were the legitimate brainchild of one man in particular, that would be Lord William Beveridge. Beveridge, an economist and pro-gressive with strong ties to the Fabian Society socialists, published in 1942 his famous *Report of the Inter-Departmental Committee on Social Insurance and Allied Services* (yes, *Beveridge Report* does sound better). The *Report* named "Five Great Evils" in society—squalor, ignorance, want, idleness, and disease—with the understanding that these would be best addressed and overcome through a gradual but systematic expansion of the State's role as the Provider of Welfare. It seemed to tap into a growing egalitarian sentiment and so, like a bottle of liquor at a frat party, the *Report* was passed around and liberally consumed.

One of the main imbibers of the Beveridge report was a Welsh fellow named Aneurin Bevan (don't ask me to explain the proliferation of "Bevs" present at the launch of the NHS). A Labour Party politician, Bevan held the position of Minister for Health from 1945 to 1951 and might best be dubbed "Beveridge's bulldog." Under the influence of his fiercely principled and unabashed socialism, the British Parliament passed two National Health Service Acts, one for England and Wales in 1946 and a second for Scotland in 1947. Bevan then fought an 18-month dispute with the resistant members of the British Medical Association before successfully gathering roughly 2,688 English and Welsh hospitals under his fatherly supervision.

I imagine too that, when it first rolled out, the incarnation of Beveridge's call for "comprehensive health and rehabilitation services" took to the streets like a recently polished Rolls Royce. But any honest onlooker today will admit that the NHS—still surviving as a source of national pride for many—is a real clunker. I say this not to offend British sensibilities but in the interests of accuracy.

CUSTOMER (DIS)SERVICE

Murray Rothbard, the famous Austrian economist, argued that the only way to maintain a monopoly is to exercise coercion—to resort to billy clubs and badges. That is essentially the business model the British have adopted, specifically with respect (or, if you ask me, disrespect) to the matter of health-care. Taxpayers contribute shares to a pool from which funds are then drawn and allocated by government administrators. What this does, however, is render the consumer of health-care services an *incidental receiver of benefits* at the point of use.

In contrast to a free market exchange, in which the patient maintains a greater level of control due to being "the payer," patients within a socialist scheme play a much more passive role. Although they may indeed pay their share of taxes and be entitled to receive something in return, by surrendering their monies to a centralized bureaucracy citizens waive their demands for individualized care. After which, they must sit hands-folded at the auction while a non-elected administrator bids for what they "need" at prices suitable to the good of the collective. (But who's wise and competent enough to judge what is good for "the collective"? And what about when the good of the many conflicts with the good of the few or the one?)

Prominent author and former prison doctor Theodore Dalrymple has first-hand experience with the unhealthy side-effects that spring up when individual patients are dismissed from the bargaining table. Mind you, Dalrymple is an avowed atheist. I am not. But that doesn't keep me from admiring things about my newly acquired acquaintance. For starters, he has a fine English accent and is well cultured, speaking fluently the language of France, where he

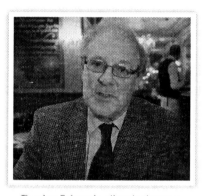

Theodore Dalrymple, otherwise knows as Dr. Anthony Daniels, a former NHS doctor and critic of Socialized health-care in the UK.

maintains a residence (however you may feel toward the French, Paris is a marvelous city). Another thing to like about him is that he is regarded by British Leftists as a curmudgeon and political Neanderthal. This is owing to opinions he holds, such as that Western intellectuals habitually relieve individuals of responsibility for their choices and thereby help cultivate an "underclass mentality" from which comes violence, promiscuity, and dependency—from drugs to welfare. In sum, they've underwritten a derelict and impoverished *way of life*. Needless to say, I wasn't surprised to find Dalrymple quite likeable.

In what turned out to be a great venue (though not our first choice), we set up across from our interviewee in a bustling Paris café. Between sips, Dalrymple recalled the sort of impatience with patients (or at least their presence) that he personally witnessed within the NHS:

> In my hospital we already had managers going around the wards... telling the doctors who they thought ought to be

discharged. They had no medical training or knowledge. But they would try and influence the doctors to discharge patients quickly... Managers are making direct clinical decisions without any clinical knowledge or experience. This is a problem, of course, wherever the person paying for the care is not the patient himself [chuckling]... But where you have one giant organization that decides everything the hazard is even greater. It's not that the hazard doesn't exist in any other system. But the more centralized a system is... the more danger there is that decisions will be taken... affecting the patient without any medical input whatsoever.

For those desiring evidence of the truly nefarious negligence that can persist when medicine is entrusted to the minions of a Single-Payer System, consider the case of Stafford Hospital (NHS), where anywhere between 400 and 1200 more patients died between 2005 and 2008 (due to substandard care) than would otherwise be expected in that type of hospital.

On February 6, 2013, barrister Robert Francis published the findings of the Mid Staffordshire NHS Foundation Trust Public Inquiry. His report stated that "patients were let down" by the Mid Staff Trust hospital and, in a press conference, Francis announced its disturbing details:

There was a lack of care, compassion, humanity, and leadership. The most basic standards of care were not observed and fundamental rights to dignity were not respected. Elderly and vulnerable patients were left unwashed, unfed, or without fluids. They were deprived of dignity and respect. Some patients had to relieve themselves in their beds when they were offered no help to get to the bathroom. Some were left in excrement-stained sheets and beds. They had to endure filthy conditions in their wards. There were incidents of callous treatment by ward staff. Patients that could not eat or drink without help did not receive it. Medicines were prescribed but not given.[2]

---

2   Robert Francis, "Statement by the Chair of the Inquiry, Robert Francis QC," at http://www. midstaffspublicinquiry.com/report; Internet; 2 August 2014.

The list went on. Although the presenter did not proceed, as I would, to reckon these tragedies as so many reasons to abandon the ideal of centrally managed health-care, he did put his finger on a crucial point:

> In short, the trust that the public should be able to place in the National Health Service was betrayed. What caused such a widespread failure of the system? This is not something that can be blamed simplistically on one policy or another, or on the failings on the part of one individual. There was an institutional culture in which the business of the system was put ahead of the priority that should have been given to the protection of the patients and the maintenance of public trust in the service.[3]

In my view, the fact that the operators of a tax-sponsored enterprise stand accountable only to other government employees and a generalized "public" largely explains why the particular individuals served may, at least eventually, figure as evils necessary for survival rather than prime motivators toward excellent customer service. Economist Murray Rothbard similarly noted, in a 1993 article, that "when government operates a service, the consumer is transmuted into a pain-in-the-neck, a 'wasteful' user-up of scarce social resources."[4]

Ever heard of Gammon's Law? Dr. Max Gammon, after studying trends and statistics within the NHS reaching back prior to the 1960s and up into the 2000s, formulated a "law of bureaucratic displacement." It describes a corporate culture in which increases in expenditures are matched by a *fall* in production through the proliferation of inflexible rules in what we call bureaucracies. Speaking at a teleconference for the Australian Doctors Fund in 2005, he contrasted the clumsy enormity of entities such as the NHS with more adaptable, light-on-their-feet organizations:

---

3   Ibid.

4   Murray Rothbard, "The Devilish Principles of Hillarycare," http://mises.org/daily/6091/The-Devilish-Principles-of-Hillarycare7.%20The%20Annoying%20Consumer; Internet; 11 October 2014. Rothbard went on to say about the Clinton health plan: "So there we have the Clintonian health future: government as totalitarian rationer of healthcare, grudgingly doling out care on the lowest possible level equally to all, and treating each 'client' as a wasteful pest. And if, God forbid, you have a serious health problem, or are elderly, or your treatment requires more scarce resources than the healthcare Board deems proper, well then Big Brother or Big Sister Rationer in Washington will decide, in the best interests of 'society,' of course, to give you the Kevorkian treatment."

Bureaucratic monsters arising among organisations [sic] whose survival depends upon their persuading customers to buy their products are sooner or later destroyed or dismembered by their competitors. However, in a protected environment, shielded from competition, a bureaucracy will grow indefinitely and approach ever more closely the black hole state, in which externally supplied resources are entirely consumed by its furious internal activity. And this is what is happening in the NHS... By contrast, within non-bureaucratic organisations [sic], continuous ad hoc procedural adjustments are made on personal initiative rather than imposed by remote directive. If successful, these local adjustments are likely to be more generally adopted. If unsuccessful, they are usually eliminated without widespread damage.[5]

This idea of a bureaucratic black hole surfaced in an episode of the 1980s BBC sitcom "Yes, Prime Minister." The PM's assistant reported to him regarding an alleged empty hospital in North London. The rumors were false, the PM learned. The hospital was not empty. In fact, there were *only* 342 administers of staff, with another 170 folks employed as porters, cleaners, laundry workers, gardeners, and cooks. When asked how many were medical staff, the assistant answered, "Oh, none of them." Due to government cutbacks, you see. Thankfully, they only had one patient, the hospital's own deputy chief administrator, who had tripped over a section of scaffolding (left up to give the appearance that the place wasn't yet open to the public) and broken his ankle.

Speaking to the dilapidated state of British hospital facilities, Dalrymple reflected on the lack of *investment* in health-care:

British hospitals are almost always jerrybuilt. Investment having come to an end in 1948... in practically all hospitals, [they] are patched together in a very unpleasant way. So that, for example, beautiful, Victorian buildings are now completely ruined by little bits that are added on to them, so that there is hardly a hospital in England that isn't a visual nightmare.

---

5   Max Gammon, "'Gammon's Law of Bureaucratic Displacement" A note from Dr Max Gammon with some quotes from Milton Friedman," at http://www.adf.com.au/archive.php?doc_id=113; Internet; 2 August 2014.

[Chuckling] And... that is a consequence of the fact that there has been no investment. And the reason there has been no investment is because of the centralization of our system.

Dalrymple's observations about the crestfallen character of NHS construction certainly resonate with me. Having both grown up in the UK and earned a degree in architecture, I have opinions on these matters.

Generally speaking, architecture is fairly resistant to short-term fads and trends. People build in ways that reflect their priorities and deeply held beliefs. Creations of stone, metal, and wood tend to stay up for a while. As such, the buildings themselves can figure as fairly faithful embodiments of deeper cultural attitudes and convictions. I can tell you that from my standpoint as a Christian the past century of British architecture clearly represents a decline of British culture. The decline is from a more glorious Christian past in the direction of a more (for the time being) secular future. This reality has shown itself in the form of modernist architectural monstrosities (such as are characteristic of the NHS) that pepper Britain.

But be careful to whom you say such things. Speaking to how the British defend the honor of the NHS as one would a spouse, Dalrymple blames a general malaise and sickly herd mentality that is preventing a proper divorce from the unattractive yet beloved health service:

> The British worship [the NHS], partly because, I think, they have very little else now to be proud of. And unfortunately they've attached their pride to something which does not merit their pride.

> There is another aspect of the... pride in the National Health Service, and that is, if conditions are uncomfortable, at least they're uncomfortable for everybody. I think the British would rather that everyone were uncomfortable than that 80% of the people were comfortable and 20% were uncomfortable. They think it's more just. In fact, it's a sign of justice, that the system is rather uncomfortable for everyone.

Some comfort is available, I suppose, if you can sit down to an old episode of "Yes, Prime Minister" and get a good laugh at how bad things are and have been for quite a while.

Daniel Hannan is someone who has a good sense of how bad things are but doesn't find it all that funny. Hannan is a forty-three year old, sharp-dressing shaper of contrarian British political opinion. Among his political and literary exploits, he has extensively publicized the positive role of markets, confronting the bureaucratic bloat and sub-standard service on display at the NHS. Consequently, he's also well acquainted with the way any serious criticism of Britain's nationalized system is stubbornly viewed by a British majority as a sort of religious impertinence.

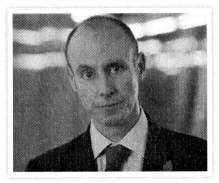

For those relatively unfamiliar with him, Hannan is a member of the European Parliament who represents South East England for the Conservative Party. A British politician, journalist, and author, Hannan was raised in Lima, Peru. He is fluent in Spanish and French and is an outspoken skeptic about

Daniel Hannan is a young, outspoken politician who specifically wanted to warn Americans against moving down the path toward increased government control of health-care.

the European Union. We met up with Hannan in Brussels, another city earning my architectural disdain. (If I may offer my own two cents, Europe's Parliament meets in an oversized steel and glass case of debased policies and spiritual emptiness. Feel free to quote me on that.)

To go with his many other notable achievements, in March 2009 a video featuring Hannan went viral on YouTube when he responded to a speech by then Prime Minister Gordon Brown with a short speech of his own, criticizing what he regarded as Brown's casual and ill-considered response to the financial crisis then erupting. Hannan was, as it were, scolding Brown for playing the robotic politician who threatens a recession with more spending and fends off a debt crisis with a new credit card.

I mention this episode because I see an important link between that line of criticism and his effort to sound an alarm about the self-perpetuating nature of a socialized bureaucracy once it's put in place. I especially appreciated his response when I asked him to talk about the zealous devotion of the British to the NHS:

People often quote Nigel Lawson, who was Margaret Thatcher's chancellor, saying that the NHS is the closest thing that the British people have to a religion. What's interesting and what's less quoted is what he said next. He said because it's treated as a religion it is impossible to reform, because the public sees these sacerdotal figures—who are the administrators and doctors in the system—against a bunch of elected politicians. And every fiber in their body... tells them to trust the people running the system rather than the politicians... That is a recipe for producer capture, for inflexibility, lack of accountability to the patients, to the customers. And that's basically been the problem right from the start.

Facing such a groundswell of religious support, it's little wonder that Hannan is eager to rouse citizens from their dogmatic slumbers:

One of the big defenders of the current healthcare system that we have—with all its anomalies and imperfections—is what Milton Friedman called "the tyranny of the *status quo*."... Our very natural human tendency is to benchmark any new proposal against existing practice and to be more frightened of change than inspired by the possibility of improvement.

These things said, he issued a strong warning to Americans who may be inclined to think they will easily be able to make a U-turn after taking a test run down the road toward collectivism:

Don't imagine that what's happened in Europe couldn't happen in the U.S. People respond to incentives. What has served to keep America prosperous and free is the institutions designed in that little miracle that happened in the old courthouse in Philadelphia. They've served the purpose which their authors intended, namely, to keep the citizen big and the government small. But if you make enough people dependent on the government, if you raise spending, and taxation, and debt to European levels, you see how long it will take before Americans start behaving and voting like Frenchmen and Greeks. There's no magic to keep the U.S. the way it is. It's not some special property in the soil, or in the water, or in the sky.

People respond to incentives. And if you switch the incentives, to make enough people want—demand—government intervention, then that's what you'll get.

Once critical mass is reached among both citizens and legislators, a socialist bureaucracy, fueled by its clientele of dependents, will behave like a runaway locomotive. Even amidst protests and cries for reform, the train is off and running.

WADING TOWARD LIVERPOOL

If you ask me, the prospect of the State extending its regulative and redistributive reach is especially menacing in the context of health-care. Doctors who seek to deal directly and compassionately with their patients will confront the fragility of life and the reality of death in a way that transcends files and statistics. In their work, they will seek both to cure and to comfort. But notice the intimate nature of this, then imagine how the *practice of health-care* and consequently *health itself* stand to be negatively impacted by the injection of government agents—remote managers uniquely shielded from risk and reward—into the business of patient care. How is this? Along with the fact that a bureaucracy has few mechanisms for adjusting to customer wants, we should focus on the dynamics of redistribution as well as the price-fixing that occurs when coercive agencies (AKA governments) become players in any market.

First, for a socialistic system to remain solvent a large number of those making deposits into the health-care fund cannot be among those withdrawing much from it. Picture a large, public swimming pool in which young, healthy people are allowed to traffic, but only at the shallow end. Also, the youths are required to make sure the spigots are running while they wade about. These represent the socialist system's financial inputs, the spots where the money is deposited. On the other end of the pool, however, it is much deeper. The people swimming there do cannonballs and splash around quite a bit. Also, on average they're a good deal more round and wrinkly. These people represent the socialist system's concentrated outputs, where the money is withdrawn to do its work. Finally, there's the lifeguard, who sits comfortably in his perch, deciding where folks can play and perhaps even whether they'll be allowed to play at all. He likes to blow his whistle and play the savior. He works for the government.

Second, whether we're talking about a fully nationalized system like the NHS or a system that grants government protection to certain "private" market participants, what we're discussing is minimizing the market share of various would-be competitors, if not keeping some out the health-care supply business altogether. In other words, we're talking about restricting supply. This restriction of supply inevitably leads to higher prices, so long as demand doesn't drop significantly. Yet higher prices are often why we're told the government must get involved in the first place. So, further efforts (coercive in nature) are made to bend costs down. This, however, drives out marginal suppliers who cannot afford to do business at the newly suppressed prices. Thus, unless the government subsidization generates a surplus on the supply side, there will be continued pressure to impose limits on what services may be dispensed and to whom.

It is, therefore, quite appropriate to describe socialized health-care as *rationed* health-care. This is not to fault the practice of rationing as such. Whereas free markets leave individuals to act in terms of their ranked values, calculating how best to express those values through trading and judicious budgeting, socialized health-care can only resort to estimating supply and demand in terms of large aggregates. As such, the country that embraces socialist medicine eliminates a profound network of signals that would otherwise be transmitted between the consumers and providers of medical goods and services. Moreover, the persistent problem of shortages that results from price-fixing and a dissipating entrepreneurship should strike us as a very undesirable scenario in the area of health-care. Indeed, government rationing of health-care services counts as an example of the sort of unhealthy competition that Michael Porter describes in his book *Redefining Health Care* as "zero sum." Rather than relying on innovation, such competitors rely on cost shifting and the limit of services to gain market share at another would-be provider's expense.

Yet, there it is. A general public demands services from the practitioners employed by Britain's NHS. Now, what to do in the socialist commonwealth when demand outstrips supply? How to respond when, for example, sickly patients outnumber the available government gurneys?

According to Dr. Patrick Pullicino, the low bed-to-patient ratio is a genuine problem and now poses a threat to the integrity of British medical practice. In June 2012, Dr. Pullicino, a consulting neurologist for the NHS, jolted attendees at a Royal Society of Medicine meeting by suggesting that prioritizing economic concerns to make space available in British hospitals constitutes a risk to patient wellness. In particular, he gained widespread media attention for sounding an alarm about something called the Liverpool Care Pathway (or LCP).

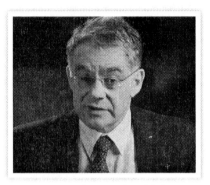

The LCP, although designed as "palliative care" with the intent of bringing comfort to patients on the edge of death, was feared to be broadly serving as a way to hasten them up to and over that edge. The Pathway falls under the Guidelines produced by the National Institute for Health and Care Excellence or NICE. Along with bearing a name a bit too similar to those of fiendish

Whistleblower, Professor Patrick Pullicino, the British neurologist who exposed a nasty side of the British NHS when he pulled back the curtains from the now infamous "Liverpool Care Pathway."

entities found in 20th century dystopian novels, such as C.S. Lewis's National Institute of Coordinated Experiments (in *That Hideous Strength*) and George Orwell's Ministry of Truth (in *1984*), Britain's NICE is tasked by the Department of Health with providing national guidelines for the use of health technology, clinical practice, public sector health-care promotion, and "social care" services. While it still flourished (as it does no longer), the LCP gave us a picture of what eventually happens when we blend a one-size-fits-all mentality with centralized rule making under the auspices of a secularized bureaucracy.

Especially powerful is Dr. Pullicino's own testimony about a patient he succeeded in removing from the Pathway. It was a story I was interested to hear when we finally got together:

> I had this elderly patient... he had a seizure disorder... This particular time he came in with a combination of pneumonia and seizures... He wasn't an easy patient from the nurses' point of view... But I was sure that he could be gradually improved over a little bit of time... with good care... And so I went off one Friday from the ward and came back on Monday and I went into his room there and I saw him just completely flat

out and I said, "Well, what's happened to this patient?"... And the relatives were in tears and they came to me and they said, "They're not giving any fluids. What's happened to him?"... When I was told that the patient had been put on the Liverpool Care Pathway I just told them they had to stop it.

In the days and weeks that followed, Dr. Pullicino oversaw the patient being nursed back to a healthier condition and returned home from the hospital. He ended up living for another 14 months before suffering another downturn that landed him on the Pathway again, where he then died.

I want to take a few moments here to talk about that patient.

These days I do quite a bit of public speaking about filmmaking. In particular, I talk quite a bit about the merits of making documentaries, as opposed to feature films. After discussing the cost advantages (documentaries tend to be significantly cheaper), I usually pause to talk about an important feature that I think set documentaries apart from fictional movies. Documentaries are lengthy, highly thematic reality dramas. The big word in there that I want to focus on is 'reality.' Rather than devise characters and stories more or less from scratch, documentarians look to discover authentic people and situations in the world in order to integrate their personalities, ideas, and stories into a work of entertaining, informative, action-inducing art—the documentary. When we reflect the world accurately, we document details of the Lord's providential designs. As Paul said, using a line from a Greek poet, "In him we live and move and have our being" (Acts 17:28).

What's even more gripping is how things sometimes come together in the very making of a film to teach us about God's supreme competence as the Director. I've found it extremely gratifying to see the complex circumstances of the stories, ideas, and people that he's sent into the path of our team. One story in particular stood out in the production of *Wait Till It's Free*.

We had wrapped up shooting in England and were bound for France, where we were to meet and interview Theodore Dalrymple. In the meantime, we stayed with my friend and former pastor, Rev. John Harding, who lives in Deal, England. We didn't guess at the time that there was any non-trivial connection between our host and the subject matter of our project.

After returning to the States from the European continent, we interviewed Professor Pullicino and learned about Sammy di Francisci—his British patient. In vain, we tried to gain, through our own efforts some connection or point of contact with the di Francisci family. The most we learned was that they lived in Deal. In passing the information on to Rev. Harding, however, I was surprised to learn that he had served as a teacher of one of the di Francisci daughters. This experience taught me again about the mystery and wisdom of Providence and reminded me that— in all our striving to connect dots and pull together the pieces of a story—God is doing His own work in and through our lives. We're

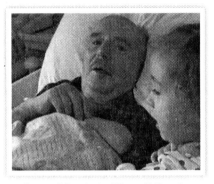

Sammy di Francisci, a UK grandfather who became ill and was placed on the LCP after being hospitalized near his home in England.

part of his dramatized reality project. The unexpected connection with Sammy's family through an older acquaintance of mine also serves as a reminder that the Triune God attends to us. We are people with *histories*. The Lord is well acquainted with where we've been, what we've done, the ways we've suffered, and where we're headed. He isn't a fly-by-night doctor who is content with a surface diagnosis or a hasty treatment plan. Christ is God with us.

This insight comes through in Sammy's story. It's not a story that I share in order to tug on the heartstrings in a morbid way. Rather, I hope that, by telling it, the Liverpool Care Pathway comes to represent the actual harm that can be done when those acting in the name of the public good—some of them doctors—swap patient care tailored to individuals for a devotion to certain established services within a system. Sammy's story should also further ingrain in us this lesson: how you pay for health-care has everything to do with the type of service that you should expect to receive.

It might not seem obvious, but I don't share the LCP story to incite indignation about how unfriendly those British nurses and doctors can be. I'm more interested in showing how people respond to incentives, particularly perverse incentives. Why, after all, would good doctors and nurses use the Pathway? In no way should we excuse individuals for their immoral choices, but no moral agent acts in a vacuum. We live and operate within the context of certain moral communities and political systems. To put it bluntly, with respect to human communities, a *system* is what emerges when the life and liberty of individuals are sacrificed on the altar of the "People's Interest." Along these lines, I found Dr. Pullicino had a keen sense of how perverse incentives encourage perverse actions, sometimes leaving individual patients to foot the bill with curtailed lives:

> There was the legal backup that supported it, there was the Pathway there, there's the pressure of beds, there's the demographics, and then, if that wasn't enough, there were actually financial incentives given to hospitals in the United Kingdom for putting people on the Pathway. And not only that, there were targets. So, they say, 'We want to get as many people on this pathway because this is the optimal way of... caring for people when they die.' So, they got set targets and, for reaching the targets, they got financial incentives... The whole thing was like a machine.

That's right. The bloated, bureaucratic stink-hole of an excuse for healthcare—the NHS—has done us the disservice of greasing the wheels toward euthanasia.

With Daniel Hannan, I don't want Americans suffering the delusion that we will be able to hopscotch over the rotten statist fruit that's presently sticking to the shoes of NHS doctors and administrators. Sadly, there's a veritable bevy of Americans who are prepared to entertain that delusion. Among them are some media heavyweights who have assisted in poisoning the well against a freed up market in medicine and health. In his film *Sicko*, for one, the renowned documentarian Michael Moore comes down hard on health insurance companies and HMOs for their rationing of procedures and treatment for the sake of financial rewards. But then he turns around and, in the next breath, praises the Clintons for their efforts in the 1990s to procure universal health coverage for all through central collection and redistribution. What Moore perhaps didn't anticipate in 2007 is that the soon-to-arrive ACA law integrates the ACO (Accountable Care Organization). In many ways following the HMO model, ACOs, while subject to the oversight of the anti-trust division of the Justice Department, continue to perpetuate *consolidation* at the expense of *competition*.

It's also worth reiterating that "Obamacare" has not been even slightly immune to the sliminess of K Street. Congressman Billy Tauzin, as Moore's film gleefully informs us, lent a helping hand in bringing down Hillarycare in 1994 right before he went to work as a powerful lobbyist for PhRMA. That is all true. But I also learned from Tim Carney that Tauzin and PhRMA threw their considerable weight behind the efforts to have the ACA law passed in exchange for protection of their own interests. Cronyism.

How exactly does narrowing the supply of health and care through restrictions and subsidies make their proffered goods and services more available and less costly to those of us who aren't filthy rich lobbyists? Good question.

We've been treated to a great deal of mischief making on the health-care front. I believe it will come back to haunt us. Remember this: when you centralize the rationing and dispensing of care for the sick and suffering—as we are in the process of doing now more than ever in this country—you place your health and life in the hands of those who are good at playing God.

Don't act surprised, therefore, when you find them doing what they're good at.

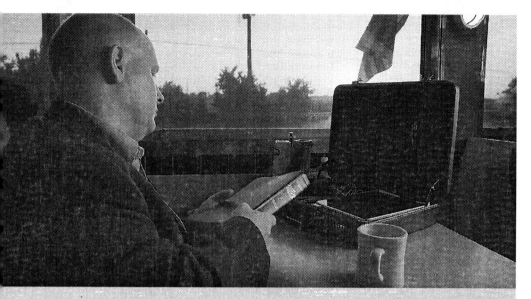

8 OUR PHILOSOPHY OF HEALTH... CARE

THE HUMAN CONDITION AND ITS IMPROVEMENT

If you empty the world of purpose, make it one of brute fact alone, you empty it... of reasons for gratitude, and a sense of gratitude is necessary for both happiness and decency. For what can soon, and all too easily, replace gratitude is a sense of entitlement. Without gratitude, it is hard to appreciate, or be satisfied with, what you have: and life will become an existential shopping spree that no product satisfies.[1]

No, these words are not to be found within the published works of a Protestant philosopher like Cornelius Van Til or Francis Schaeffer. They appear in an article by the atheist doctor from the previous chapter, Theodore Dalrymple, in which he further states that to regret [Christian] religion is to regret "our civilization and its monuments, its achievements, and its legacy."[2]

---

1 Theodore Dalrymple, "What the New Atheists Don't See," at http://www.city-journal.org/html/17_4_oh_to_be.html; Internet; 2 August 2014.

2 Ibid.

I'm writing this book in English and intend it to address twenty-first century Americans. When I talk about health-care, therefore, I'm doing so within the stream of the Christian West and its secular decline over at least two centuries. I make these remarks to help us reflect on a broader historical and philosophical matrix in which this book participates. More specifically, I wish to convey that "health-care" is not itself a culturally, morally, or religiously neutral concept. To have a concept of "health-care" is to have a concept of at least certain aspects of the human condition and, presumably, what counts as threats as well as improvements to that condition. And to have a concept of the human condition and its improvement is to take what amounts to a religious viewpoint.

From the first, we need to think this through Christianly. Because the Lord "giveth to all life, and breath, and all things," it is fitting to capitalize on the raw materials he supplies and the causal structures he imposes, while giving him thanks and praise for his continuous generosity. On one side of the coin, Christians acknowledge that they are members of a fallen race moving about on a sin-stained earth. On the other side, they acknowledge their need for healing and show the Triune power behind their faith when they trust the Physician and Provider and take the bread and wine He prescribes. Moreover, the redeeming work of Christ embraces not some mere spiritual stratosphere but the entire creation.

In reference to a philosophy of medicine and health, the late R.J. Rushdoony discussed some features of Christian thought that profoundly shape how we talk about these issues and what we expect from physicians. Two deserve to be mentioned here. First, Christians believe that the heavens and earth are governed by divine providence. A personal Lord works his purposes not only through the stars but also through the intricacies of the human body. Second, within that same understanding, the physician is not merely a manipulator of localized "physics." In addition to tending to the body, those to whom we have *entrusted* ourselves in Western Christendom have been called "doctors" (which, in Latin, means *teacher*, from *docere*, to teach). They are personal agents who tend with concern. Patients (and doctors) are integrated persons or body-souls, responsible to walk before God and be holy in all manner of living (I Peter 1:15).

FLUKEIAN HABITS OF THOUGHT

But here, amidst the worldly air we breathe, the concept of *teleology* (or divine purpose) frequently and habitually gets traded for the idea that man is a strictly material, mechanical being. The would-be autonomous man's hope, in parallel fashion, is not set on the Creator or rooted in the Three-in-One who will raise up bodies for a Last Day evaluation. His expectations must naturally be more provincial and pragmatic. Without trying to multiply insults, I'd wager that the thoughts of the secular man on the street rarely range far beyond: what sort of insider knowledge can keep me from having to face death or even from having to think about it? If he is prone to replace divine governance with a deified human government, perhaps he thinks: how can I get others to pay for my medical bills?

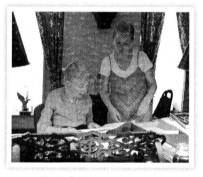

Phyllis Schlafly has fought the feminist agenda since the Equal Rights Amendment in the early 70s.

This does seem to be the way of things. As individuals, families, church bodies, and local communities have in the past century increasingly refrained from bearing their own and each other's burdens, some folks have been happy to see that. If they could, those I have in mind would remove social and institutional reminders of God's revealed will for human life. An important part of that project involves a "replacement theology," in which the State stumbles along to shoulder burdens formerly assumed at a local and spiritual level. Phyllis Schlafly, whom I consider a matriarch of American conservatism for the past forty years, spoke to a crucial aspect of this when I asked her what she thinks motivates people like Barack Obama and Kathleen Sebelius to so strongly back the abortion lobby:

> Well, the liberals and the feminists and the socialists really look upon the traditional family as an enemy, a political enemy of what they're for. So, they want to break up the family. The only way you could have limited government is to have intact, nuclear families that really manage their own lives, take care of their own children, and so forth... What Obama's tried to do is to [add to] the percentage of people who are dependent for

their daily living on the government. In fact, it's approaching almost half of our society now. And if you're dependent on government for some of your living expenses, you're very agreeable to... doing what you're being told [to do].

As my earlier films emphasized, the fruit of a godless quest for autonomy—particularly relating to sexuality—is plentifully scattered around the ground we walk on.

In case you haven't noticed, sin can be expensive, especially when someone else (other than the beneficiary) is footing the bills. The Sandra Fluke story serves as a recent illustration. In February 2012, Fluke, a Georgetown law student, argued before a panel of House Democrats that Georgetown University should be forced by law to offer a health care plan that pays for birth control drugs. She complained that 40% of Georgetown Law's female population suffers financially due to lack of coverage for contraceptives and insisted that the demand for a steady diet of birth control pills (which typically include an abortifacient fail-safe mechanism) should be met, in spite of the Catholic school's moral opposition to artificial birth control as such (not to mention abortion).

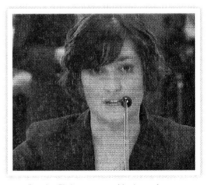

This violent wielding of a sense of entitlement should emblazon upon our brains at least three things.

First, the moral attitudes and actions of individuals in a society shape the way health-care is understood, financed, and administered. If you no longer view man as made in

Sandra Fluke appeared before a house committee to complain about the problem of not receiving insurance coverage for birth control through her Roman Catholic college.

God's image, if you remove magistrates from under the divine jurisdiction, and if you place the State at the disposal of those abandoned to their animal impulses, then you will suffer a perverted concept of healthiness. One's idea of *man*, indeed, drives one's vision of man's *thriving* and policies promoted pursuant that vision. I don't think it's just a weird coincidence, for example, that Britain's NHS features a Gender Identity Clinic, where an adolescent diagnosed with "gender dysphoria" can receive hormone treatments to suppress his or her natural, pubescent development and, if one graduates to adulthood—lo and behold—persuaded that an expertly performed genital mutilation is in order, well, the taxpayers really sort of owe it to him, her, or whatever. When you build Frankenstein, don't be surprised when that soul-less monster starts haunting you.

Second, never mind the wayward and beggaring libidos that Fluke would unleash upon the taxpayers. She represents a *modus operandi* to which increasing numbers in the land are becoming acclimated. Think for a moment of how "health-care" seems to occupy a spot toward the top of her expectations in life. The Buddhists might say she suffers an attachment to it. I see it as an idol, but also as one thread within a larger, tragic tapestry of what I'll call health-care hubris. What I have in mind here relates to a line of thinking drawn out by medical ethicist and retired MD, Edward Payne. As one who has sought to think God's thoughts after him about the practice and practitioners of medicine, Payne believes that thoughtful Christians should have a much lower estimate of the concrete, empirical successes of modern health-care than is common.

In particular, he calculates that when the 1.21 million abortions that occur each year in the U.S. (roughly one-third of the total number of deaths) are taken into account, the average lifespan of an American suddenly drops to below age 50. It also bears mentioning that abortions are routinely performed not by "quacks" but by supposedly bona fide (i.e., licensed) physicians (who are, incidentally, subsidized by the insurance dollars of Christians). This observation should at least tell us that the healthiness of a nation does not consist in the pharmaceuticals, instruments, or credentials it has for possessions. It turns out, rather, that health and well-being have at least as much to do with how one lives and treats life as they do with accessing the latest wonder drugs or imaging techniques. Let us not discount, therefore, the Law of God when it comes to judging how well we promote and maintain life and health.

Third, Fluke's apparent disregard for the survival of both property rights and defenseless infants showcases the coercive, deathward spiral in which we are caught. On one hand, we are witnessing strides away from the voluntary acquisition and distribution of medical services. The paint is still fresh on the ACA's punitive tax on the uninsured, the current Chief Executive having splattered it against the already messy background of wealth transfers called Medicare and Medicaid. On the other hand, we are also witnessing a ratcheting up of coercive constraints on the supply of medical services.

This ought to concern anyone who doesn't wish to have his medical destiny determined by "civil servants" who've been trained and paid to serve the system, frequently at the expense of individual patients.

POWER RELIGION AND THE RATIONING OF PATIENT CARE

In his book *Moses and Pharaoh*, Dr. Gary North distinguishes something he calls *power religion*. Power religion is a faith that expresses itself whenever power and wealth are sought and maintained without a proper acknowledgment of Christ's ethical jurisdiction over all of life. Sadly, a tug-a-war between this sort of humanism and what North calls *dominion religion*—an approach to piety and politics characterized by its commitment to God's supreme Law-Word—has from many angles been lost through compromises with a Gnostic sort of faith that he calls *escapist religion*. What I want to do is call us to re-engage our spiritual opponent and tighten our grip. Christ has been given all authority in heaven and earth (Matthew 28:18). It's again time to resist actively those who think we can get our money for nothin' and our health (or at least some semblance of it) for free (AKA through appropriation and inflation). For, in their failing efforts, the proponents of State power—being culpably ignorant of Christ's ethical authority—are not apt to resign the reins of control. More likely, they will, wherever and whenever they can, reassert and expand their might and influence.

Jerri Lynn Ward is quite familiar with the path that power religion paves for those determined to walk it and she regrets that we seem to be straying further along that route. As an attorney out of Austin, Texas, Ward has advocated since 2006 for numerous patients who, for one reason or another, are labeled by their physicians as "futile care" recipients and threatened with the withdrawal of life-sustaining treatments. She discerns two separate motivations that account for why some patients, especially those dependent on the government to bankroll their care, are being hurried toward hospice:

> It's two-fold. One, something very bad is happening in the
> area of medical ethics... Doctors are being raised up in such a

manner that they actually think some life is not worth living...
The other motivation is money. Because... essentially, this is
the precursor of the rationing of health-care. Many of the
people who I've helped have been either on Medicare or
Medicaid. And, of course, there's an impetus there when we're
talking about government dollars... to try to save money. But
I have noticed that oftentimes they don't start up the futility
protocols until that person is near the end of their insurance
policy or end of... number of days of Medicare or end of
Medicaid benefits.

Her experiences have not encouraged Ward to fight for expanded financial
inputs into the existing welfarism the U.S. has in place. What they *have*
done is acquaint her with the negative effects lying in store for patients
when market regulators and wealth redistributors are inserted between
them and their care providers.

Not all of the effects are as dramatic as the removal of respirators and
feeding tubes. Obamacare, we should know by now, is about giving. Under
the colorfully lit ACA tree, we find ACOs. These represent a repackaging
of the HMO model—"Accountable Care Organizations." As John Goodman
explains in *Priceless: Curing the Healthcare Crisis*, ACOs will resemble HMOs
in offering doctors financial incentives for withholding care but with the
added bonus of placing them "under intense pressure to practice medicine
according to guidelines written by people you will never meet or see."[3]
These are stockings full of treats. Welcome to a world where Washington's
guidelines and checklists are master to their physician servants. A second
"big brotherly" feature of the ACA is the full flowering of HIPAA—the
Health Insurance Portability and Accountability Act—through the funding
of a federal data bank containing the medical records of those herded into
the narrow networks of participating providers.

All of this is done, of course, in the name of securing health-care for all.
But you can't get something for nothing. One of the costs of this "blessing"
of mandated coverage under a federally restricted range of providers will be
a limited availability of quality care. There are a number of reasons why we
should expect this.

3 John Goodman, "The HMO in Your Future," at http://townhall.com/columnists/johncgood-man/2012/06/23/the_hmo_in_your_future/page/full; Internet; 2 August 2014.

First, in order to compete or survive in the marketplace, marginal players will be increasingly forced to join larger hospitals or networks. This consolidation trend will tend to cut against quality, as it will mean fewer alternatives—say, fewer options from which to choose when seeking a doctor offering a second opinion. If Dr. B belongs to the same provider network as Dr. A, how likely is it that Dr. B will place a check on Dr. A's diagnosis and treatment plan by offering an alternative one, perhaps at a lesser price?

A second way in which quality stands to suffer relates to what Ward calls "check box" medicine. The security of having a government-protected job (so long as they check those boxes!) will surely attract people to the medical profession. But the replacement of the market's carrot and stick (profits and losses, both monetary and social) with even greater regulatory burdens will prevent many bright, innovative people from entering or staying in the medical profession although they otherwise might.

These so-called reforms taking place are not, then, moving us closer to making doctors more accountable to their patients. Rather, we're inducing the supposed caregivers to serve a system—everybody in general and nobody in particular. Under those conditions, individual patients will not be able to trust a medically trained professional to represent their interests in the face of a government lackey eager to roll them toward the exit door.

From a Christian standpoint, these socio-economic developments are especially troubling when it's understood that those eager to dispense with a biblical understanding of *liberty and tyranny* aren't prone to hold very tenaciously to a biblical understanding of *life and death*. It's at this point that opposition to State-managed rationing of health-care boils over into a concern that those who are politically marginalized—e.g., unwanted infants, comatose patients, and the chronically expensive elderly—will be the first ones to have their care curtailed or removed entirely.

I asked James Lansberry, Executive Vice President of Samaritan Ministries, to talk about the politicization of health-care and he had this to say:

> When you look at health-care and you look at our culture, you have to look back to the Scriptures... what God says: "Those who hate me love death." And the triple crown of death in health-care is eugenics, abortion, and euthanasia. And we oppose all of those, as Christians. We have to oppose all of

those. But those are a part of what the government is going to be active in. If you look at the most heinous crimes that have been committed over the past 300 years, all of those have been government-sponsored, whether it be Nazi Germany, Stalin... any major campaign against people. Those were not committed by free people. They were committed by totalitarian states.

He then discussed something known as the IPAB (or Independent Payment Advisory Board). The IPAB is a fifteen-member agency created by the ACA and assigned the fool's errand of achieving savings in Medicare in ways that leave coverage and quality unaffected. Unlike its predecessor, MedPAC (Medicare Payment Advisory Commission), the IPAB does not act in a mere advisory role. While their actions are subject to being overruled by Congress, the panel members have the power to change the Medicare program and a congressional supermajority is required to trump their decisions. Little wonder that even some Democrats fear that the IPAB grants what Keynesian economist Paul Krugman wished for when he said that, in order to keep and manage Medicare, what will be necessary is "death panels and sales taxes."[4]

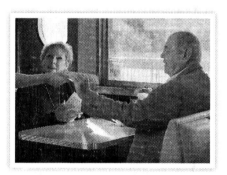

Health-care rationing is a harsh reality that those among the Baby Boom generation will increasingly face.

This is indeed a scary development. But the consistency of someone like Krugman, who is prepared to articulate his faith in central planning, helps drive home the point that the way one pays for some thing or service profoundly affects how that thing or service is received (or whether it is received at all).

Krugman the Keynesian does have a point though. Capital is finite. Because the demand for services will sometimes outpace the means of supplying services, the allocators will occasionally be forced to maintain solvency by prorating those services that are financed, imposing restric-

---

4   Paul Krugman, "Death Panels and Sales Taxes," at http://krugman.blogs.nytimes.com/2010/11/14/death-panels-and-sales-taxes/?_php=true&_type=blogs&_r=0; Internet; 2 August 2014.

tions on the services that are provided, or both. This is called rationing, as I've said before, and we all do it. Some kind of "economizing" of health-care is unavoidable in any context and is not objectionable in itself. What is objectionable is the threatened loss of personal dignity (and perhaps even health and life) that results when decisions about the propriety of a treatment or procedure are left to a remote (or even nearby) bureau of planners.

Tom Kendall, a general practitioner from Greenville, S.C. and the current President of AAPS, agrees that the collectivizing (and thereby politicizing) of health-care poses a mounting risk to the well-being of both patients and their families:

> The consequences of a politicized health-care system... the fruit of the principles that drive that politic will be born out in the context of disease, treatment, health considerations, family... I am a family physician and the focus of my attention is "how does this disease process affect the family?" How can we help this family have a response to disease that is going to result in healing and restoration, rather than singling out a diagnosis and focusing upon the cost of that diagnostic... current procedural code... to get compensated? The most important thing is not getting paid for a procedure. The most important thing is seeing what's most important for the patient.

What this calls for, he believes, is a principled stand, by doctors especially, on the side of liberty and free exchange in the world of health and health-care:

> The medical profession is one of the noblest professions of mankind. I'm so grateful that God allowed me to be a physician. But with that privilege comes great responsibility. And it's only within the last several years that I've recognized the great need of that jurisdictional privilege that I have to work to preserve liberty... As a physician, I've taken on the role of trying to understand how best to go forward with the preservations of our liberty. Talk is important. But actually working out the details of that liberty in the patient-physician relationship...

and the understanding of how to go forward with that is a big endeavor. It's a major work right now.

Thankfully, Dr. Kendall is not alone in that endeavor. There are still doctors out there who are unwilling to have their patient loyalties compromised and some are going out of their way to prove it.

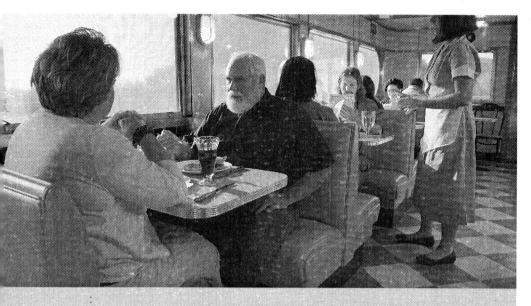

9 : BACK TO THE PATIENTS

The title of this chapter is meant as a word play. *In the beginning*, we'd like to say, doctors were upright, dedicated to their patients. Due to distracting financial influences and regulatory burdens introduced by third parties, however, they appear to have sought out various devices. If we're talking metaphors, which we are, the trend for a good portion of the past century has been for doctors to *turn their backs* on the patients. Today, this is sadly, quite literally, too often the case. As the fearful subjects of technocratic coding regimes that control medical billing, doctors today are increasingly more likely to have their heads buried in a computer during a consultation than turned toward their patient.

But let's not rest on a complaint about that. There are reasons for optimism after all. Here I'd like to talk about two of those reasons, Juliette Madrigal-Dersch ("Madrigal" for short) and G. Keith Smith. Madrigal and Smith are physicians who, both in how they service consumers and in how they market their services, are turning back to their patients.

ALWAYS A DOCTOR

Whereas, some doctors will recall knowing that they were going into medicine and perhaps even a particular sub-field by the age of ten, that wasn't the case for Juliette Madrigal. She'd finished college and begun a career in sales by the time she first caught the doctoring bug, but once she did, it changed her for good:

> Originally, I was an advertising major and I went to New York and did advertising for a year. And when I was there one of my friends was an EMT. So... we were first on the scene of an accident and he grabbed all his stuff, went out and took care of the patient. And I was absolutely blown away... From then on I thought, "I have to do this. This is the neatest thing ever."

The sudden flush of enthusiasm didn't really cool down either. Rather, it persisted and matured as she went from sneaking into medical conferences during business trips, to working as a volunteer in the ER, to specializing in internal medicine and pediatrics, to opening her own practice in a town not too far west of Austin, Texas.

Juliette, or "Jules," is an attractive, young, friendly doctor. She also has an outstanding ability to speak boldly for her cause: medical liberty. I remember the first time we met. During the 2012 election, I was doing short, on-the-fly interviews for a pro-life cause. I was at an AAPS conference and asked to

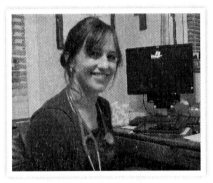

Jules (as her patients call her) runs a cash-only family practice in Marble Falls, Texas.

interview Jules (president of AAPS at the time). After the interview, we were getting into an elevator and heading back to the conference when several firemen joined us on an emergency call. It turned out that a doctor at the conference had suffered a heart attack.

What struck me (and still sticks in my mind) was how swiftly and unhesitatingly Jules leaped into action. Once we reached the scene, she rushed towards the doctor and quickly started giving chest compression.

I realized in those moments the importance of competent doctors. They do things that other people don't know how to do or, at the very least, are unwilling to do. While Jules was working on her fallen colleague, I did what a documentary filmmaker would probably be expected to do in such a situation. I stood as far away as possible and observed the dramatic, unfolding scene. The event reminded me that a good deal of personal fortitude and professional understanding separates a physician from a civilian like me. The physician generally possesses a great deal of both factual and practical knowledge along with the ability to apply that knowledge with grace and confidence. Needless to say, I'm constantly humbled when I meet people like this. They actually save lives.

Jules is no exception. Dr. Madrigal, however, is notable for more than her professional abilities, enthusiasm, and enjoyment of her job. For one, she doesn't view being a doctor as merely her profession. She views it as her calling. This appears, at least partially, to trace to an older style doctor that served her family when she was a girl:

> Well, I am very, very blessed and very luck to have the patients
> I have. But the way I set up this model and the way I started
> my practice was... not new. It was actually based on the doctor
> who took care of us growing up. If we were sick, he would stop
> by the house and see what was wrong with us. My mom would
> call him and he would say, "Oh, this is what it is" and he would
> take care of us.

Her experience witnessing this personalized approach helps shed light not only on the close bond she has with her patients but also on her thoughts about the proper nature of the transaction between doctor and patient.

Touching the latter, the "model" she mentions relates to the fact that she's taken a path less traveled in how she "does" medicine. And it appears to have made all the difference. After some time in the profession, Dr. Madrigal decided she would no longer accept government funds, having previously refused to get mixed up with pre-paid health coverage in the form of insurance. She thereby converted her practice to a cash-only operation.[1] "Conversion" is a good way of putting it, too. It undoubtedly takes a kind of religious conviction and confidence to break free of the system. There's another word—system. Isn't a *system* just the opposite of what practitioners in the realm of health-care should be about? To me, such talk too easily smacks of an assembly of robotic bits of clockwork moving in

---

1   For a scholarly look at the inflationary effects of third-party involvement in health-care and related information, see Maureen J. Buff and Timothy D. Terrell, "The Role of Third-Party Payer in Medical Cost Increases," http://www.jpands.org/vol19no3/buff.pdf; *Journal of American Physicians and Surgeons* Vol. 19, No. 2 (Summer 2014) 75-79; Internet; 30 October 2014.

lockstep. Not to speak badly of good order, but in addition to organization a person wants warmth and concern from his or her doctor.

I spoke earlier about how the chore of storing and converting records constitutes a relative drain on the resources of health-care providers. Included in this business is the chore of becoming thoroughly conversant in what are known as ICD codes, a sort of icing on the cake served up by the Administrative Collective. ICD stands for International Statistical Classification of Diseases and Related Health Problems, a maze of ciphers issued by the World Health Organization. In the United States, one comes under the oversight of the codes by agreeing to take Medicare or Medicaid patients. Any outfit doing so then becomes a node within the Electronic Data Interchange (EDI) under the auspices of Title II of HIPAA, which requires "the establishment of national standards for electronic health care transactions and national identifiers for providers, health insurance plans, and employers."[2] For seasoned Star Trek fans, this is roughly equivalent to joining the Borg, a single, collective mind (or "hive") that assimilates smaller, less well-armed space travelers.

That last bit may come across as neo-Luddite hyperbole. But it's pretty well in keeping with Dr. Madrigal's thoughts on the subject, and it has much more to do with serving individuals than with some supposed aversion to computers:

> Those codes reduce patients and illnesses just to... a series of numbers. So, for one, I think it's very dangerous to reduce a person to a number. It gets rid of the doctor-patient relationship and makes somebody be a... code... It really puts a barrier to care and to seeing the patient as a real person.

She thus recognizes the extensive harm done by socialized medicine's tendencies to dictate our health-care decisions by formula. Along these lines, the energy and resources required to access, interpret, and apply the ICD codes simultaneously diverts attention away from patient particularities and discourages some doctors from taking patients eligible for government benefits:

---

2 "Health Insurance Portability and Accountability Act," http://en.wikipedia.org/wiki/Health_Insurance_Portability_and_Accountability_Act; Wikipedia; Internet; 6 January 2015.

The thing about these codes is... they're used to punish doctors who don't do things correctly. If you put the wrong code on something... for example, there's one code for someone who's bit by a parrot. There's a separate code for someone's who's bitten by a macaw [disgusted eyeroll]. Okay? So, if I accidentally don't know the difference between a parrot and a macaw, then it's a... crime that I picked the wrong code. So... if they audit me, they can refuse to pay me for seeing that patient and they can actually review all my charts and say, "Well, you did this twice, so we think that 25% of your people you've seen you've probably coded wrong, too. So, we're gonna just decide and take all that money away..." That's another way that Medicare keeps doctors from really being able to take care of their patients. And it keeps doctors from wanting to take Medicare and from *wanting* to take care of those Medicare-aged people.

Tiring of all the silliness, Dr. Madrigal hit a breaking point. But it wasn't a resentment of those visiting her for care that prompted her exit from the system. It was precisely the opposite. A mindset well-attuned to patient idiosyncrasies led her to alter the way in which she accepted payment for services and to eliminate certain *sources* of payment—namely, any third party.

Isn't that interesting? In seeking to provide physician care tailored to patient individuality, this doctor thought it best to radically adjust the form of reimbursement she is willing to accept. I consider this a feather in the cap of the idea that how something is paid for has a terrific shaping influence on *what kind of something* will be delivered.

It's also arguable that her choice to forego all third party payers has made Madrigal more, not less, effective in providing charitable service than when she was bound to the government's confiscatory kindness:

I'm a cash-only clinic... I'm not responsible to an insurance company. I'm not responsible to the government. I'm only responsible to the patient. Plus, in doing so, I can do... whatever I want! We give a discount to teachers and preachers. We see foster kids for free. We see missionary kids for free a lot of the time. We see people who have cancer absolutely for free.

It's not just her charitable service that's refreshing. The more intimate interface characterizing a cash-for-service (and sometimes barter) exchange struck me as having its own positive influence on the health of Dr. Madrigal's patients. People are not kept at arm's distance through the mediation of codes and so tend to place greater value on the service provided because they are now more directly minding the details of their health-care through direct monetary exchange.

As Austrian school economists have taught, when person A exchanges Q with person B for R, person A is saying, "I value R more than I value Q" and person B is saying, "I value Q more than I value R." This expresses what is known as *quid pro quo*—"something for something."[3] However, the involvement of third parties tends to muddy the water between payment and goods or services received. This is because the third parties are also being paid for facilitating and financing the exchange. The doctor quite indirectly answers to the patient's desires. The insurance company competes at least in some measure with the doctor for the patient's approval. Going to "cash-only" means a clarified understanding of what is being exchanged for what and goes along with an expected open communication between the two parties.

One sees this born out in Dr. Madrigal's experience with her clients. Both ideologically and practically, she repudiates continual monitoring by Uncle Sam and the overly clinical bedside manner encouraged by it:

> If you have time and government's not involved... if you have time to speak with your patients, you'll learn almost everything you need to know. On the other hand, there are a lot of things that aren't medical. If you have somebody whose husband recently died and she has a stomachache and a headache and feels nauseated and is tired all the time, if you have time, you can sort out that that's probably depression. That doesn't need a CT scan... or an MRI or all those things. You just need to listen to the patient and spend time with the patient and know who they are and what's going on.

---

3   For a clear explanation of the Austrian understanding of how unequal valuations of goods and services make possible *equitable exchanges*. Gary M. Galles, "Understanding 'Quid Pro Quo," https://www.mises.org/daily/6934/Understanding-Quid-Pro-Quo; Internet; 23 October 2014.

What she's really talking about is treating patients as *whole people with histories*. What's odd about this is exactly nothing, except for how it clashes with the bland materialism encountered on the road toward the USB— United Statist Bureaucracy. On that road, the patient lines up (due to shortages), picks a number, and prepares to be treated as an assembly of parts, one or more of which may be suffering a defect. Things obviously do go wrong with parts of the body, but they are parts of the *body*. Humans are also greater than the sum of their physical organs. Greater attention to that reality, however, does not come by way of a federally mandated insurance:

> Only *people* can care for each other. But... Obamacare, there is no *care* in it. It's just a lot of numbers and regulations and fees and tables. It's not actually caring for each other. And that can only be done one-on-one... one person to another person. And when you take that out of it, it's *not* health-care anymore. It's simply medicine. And medicine is helpful but it doesn't cure people like health-care does.

If she's right—and I think she is—the efforts of politicians to "reform" health-care will not be effective unless they enable doctors to understand and walk alongside their patients as whole persons. What this looks like is politicians amputating themselves and their bureaucratic underlings from the medical marketplace. They are superfluous appendages.

Don't hold your breath waiting for that to happen. You'll end up passing out (and require a visit to the ER). But I digress. Anyway, one would probably do better to look for positive changes in the health-care arena arising from the actions of individuals and private companies who seek a more consumer-driven market.

A DIFFERENT KIND OF BUSINESS

Dr. G. Keith Smith is another doctor who is doing good in the provision of health-care without being dim-witted about it. Smith is an anesthesiologist of over twenty years as well as a co-founder and managing partner of the Surgery Center of Oklahoma in Oklahoma City.

It's sad to say, but Keith Smith is something of a cultural anomaly (like one of those rare events that can occur at the sub-atomic level). With the exception of some doctors I met through AAPS, and perhaps a handful of others, who certainly include Smith, a physician's license too often tends to be affixed at the neck like a set of dog tags. It too often means that this or that medical professional is owned by the system. The system I have in mind consists of hulking hospitals, interloping insurers, and gargantuan government programs. Through controls placed on market participation, these parties succeeded in *cartelizing* large facets of the health-care industry. One consequence of this is that there are terrific (and by that I mean *terrible*) incentives, inducing doctors to display loyalty to the various third parties rather

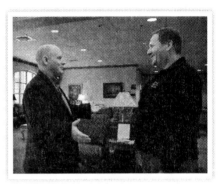

Dr. Keith Smith runs a physician-managed surgery center in Oklahoma City, Oklahoma.

than their patients. The benefits for those willing to be collared include what I'll call a "centrally protected" income and status. In other words, there are considerable perks for those willing to play the game.

Facing these grim facts, it's a delight when you find a doctor that is so radically opposed to playing the game. Keith Smith is such a doctor. He chose to skip the status quo way of doing business and instead to incline his ear the interests of the Market (patient). Motivated largely by his views on liberty, he has been willing to break the rules or, as it were, rewrite them. Upon meeting, he and I quickly realized that we shared some important common ground. In particular, we both share a keen interest in economics, especially the Austrian brand associated with names such as Carl Menger, Ludwig von Mises, Murray Rothbard, and Joseph Salerno. In Keith's case, his economic interests and beliefs are concretely displayed in the enterprises he's undertaken within his field of expertise.

Smith's Surgery Center has gained national media attention in recent years for the exceptional and efficient service its doctors provide and also for engaging in an unusual and offensive practice: honest pricing. By placing the Center's management under the direction of the doctors themselves, by refusing to take federal payment for services, by minimizing third-party involvement, and by marketing in a way that's rigorously

BACK TO THE PATIENTS

transparent about prices, Smith and company go on the offensive in at least two respects. First, they "stick it to the man," exposing the obscure and obscene out-of-pocket expenses that too often confront patients due to the "price opacity" practiced by corporate interlopers (e.g., giant insurers and hospitals). Second, they bless consumers directly by providing services at a comparably low rate and *indirectly* by equipping those familiar with the Center's high-value, low-cost reputation to negotiate prices with other providers of the same type of services. Thereby, they furnish consumers with *leveraging power*.

As such, the Surgery Center embodies a commitment to liberty. It also embodies a desire to advocate on behalf of patients—promoting a doctor-patient relationship free from outside financial and political contaminants.

Turning our attention back to Dr. Smith, his progress toward medical entrepreneurship took place gradually. Early in his career he participated in the Medicare system, but he later departed due to the paltry sums he was receiving:

> I finished my training in 1990 and came to Oklahoma City, hoping to do mostly cardiac anesthesia, even though I was trained to do pediatric anesthesia as well. Both those aspects of my practice grew very quickly. Medicare, in 1992, decided to slash payment for cardiac anesthesia services so low that I began to think that I needed to... walk away from that. They cut the price for that again in 1993 and the last cardiac anesthetic that I did was six hours long and I was paid $278. The last Medicare "total knee" that I did, I was paid $78 for that anesthetic. So I walked away from Medicare and began to have some real philosophical issues with taking that money anyhow.

From there, his pragmatic disenfranchisement with Medicare payments grew into a more principled ethical critique of coercive wealth redistribution:

> One day it occurred to me that I really had no claim on the property of my neighbor for a service that I rendered to someone across town that my neighbor didn't even know. When the person across town, to whom I'd given this service, likely could've afforded the service. So, I began seeing taking that

money as... theft, to put it real bluntly... The government doesn't have any money, after all, that they didn't first take from someone else at gunpoint.

This translated into a wholesale refusal to deal with Washington as a market participant:

So, I just decided I was not going to deal with them anymore. I would not let them leverage me. I would not count on future revenue from them. I would not write my congressman and lobby for more money... I would just act as if they didn't exist.

He had undergone a philosophical paradigm shift.

Not too long after that, Dr. Smith and his friend and fellow anesthesiologist, Dr. Steven Lantier, both dissatisfied with the level of service at their hospital and disturbed by a culture in which administrators bullied surgeons, planned to set out on their own.

In 1997, this led them to partner in the purchase of a mismanaged surgery center, hoping to do a different kind of business. They were entering the world of entrepreneurial medicine and they were doing it armed with at least two fundamental commitments. First, they would practice what Smith calls "price honesty," not quoting one thing and demanding another or surprising clients with fees that remained hidden until the services are rendered and payment is expected. Second, they would refuse to accept government payments for services. According to their calculations, they could undercut the prices charged by their competitors while delivering high quality care.

Within six months of opening up shop, their more optimistic expectations were already bearing fruit. By November 1997, Smith and Lantier received confirmation that their quoted prices were often a tenth of the alleged basement prices which local non-profit hospitals were "poor-mouthing" and claiming as the cause of financial distress. Within four years, the startup grew enough to require a new facility, one large enough to house the upsized staff and operation.

Since then, the Surgery Center of Oklahoma has proven a boon to patients, many of whom otherwise would face the likely prospect of paying huge insurance premiums or shackling themselves to exorbitant debt to finance an operation. By offering world-class care at such favorable prices to the consumer, the Surgery Center's doctors also reaped some monetary benefits. That's as it should be. As individuals and corporations are discouraged from gaining un-fair advantage by lining political pockets, the forces of supply and demand will work toward greater equilibrium. The economic land-scape will be perceived less as a *zero sum game*, in which one party's gains (or losses) exactly correspond to another party's losses (or gains). Rather, consumers will tend to reward those who best serve them. Suppliers, realizing this, will return the favor by improving quality and lowering prices in order to attract customers away from com-peting outfits. The result is a higher standard of living in the shape of cost savings and improved quality. The community wins.

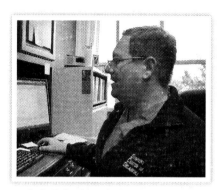

Dr. Keith Smith's website offers pure price transparency. You can go click on a link and find out exactly the cost for any operation.

Consistent with the way he runs his business, Dr. Smith is an out-spoken defender of a free market in health-care:

> There are not very many examples of the free market in health-care in the United States. But lasik surgery and plastic surgery are definitely two. In both cases, you see prices fall and the quality soar. But even if the price stays the same, the quality goes up. The value proposition is improved. I believe the reason health-care is so expensive in the United States is not a *failure* of the free market but an *absence* of a free market.

Keith even has a blog, where he regularly sounds off in support of free market principles within the medical domain.[4]

Smith identifies the consolidation of industry as a "smoking gun" for corruption and bribery—K Street activities—and views the *Unaffordable Care Act* as a further elaboration on that theme. But before we think

---

4   G. Keith Smith, http://surgerycenterofoklahoma.tumblr.com; Internet; 2 August 2014.

Obamacare is the only spooky bogeyman in the room, he would warn to us about other culprits.

Included among them is, one, the uncompensated care system (or "scam" as he puts it), whereby "non-profit" hospitals are able to gain massive government subsidies after reporting losses (based on juiced numbers). In general, non-profit hospitals are able to receive tax-sourced compensation for services rendered for the poor and uninsured. This basically creates a perverse incentive that some of the less scrupulous corporate officers use to gain advantage. They follow their noses and quite deliberately hand higher bills to those less able to pay. Yes, you read that correctly. Indeed, there are some nonprofits that are, across the board, charging greatly in excess of what insurers are willing to pay for goods or services. This allows hospital corporate heads to report fictional losses to the government and receive subsidies, without the benefit of competitive price signals determining what they charge insurers and cash-pay patients. This phenomenon help account for why something like a box of gauze can be priced by multiple factors higher at a "nonprofit" than it would be at your local CVS Pharmacy.[5]

A second culprit is the CON game or Certificate of Need. Rep. Robert Lynn of Alaska has suggested that a better name for these would be Certificates of Monopoly, as that is essentially what they are. There are both state and federal statutes that first require those seeking to establish a health-care facility to seek and acquire the blessing of a regulative agency to do so. This permission comes in the form of a Certificate of Need. Apparently assuming that government employees occupy a cool, neutral place and are eminently familiar with the best interests of "the community," we allow bureaucrats to shush noisy consumers and stifle their servants on the supply side. Meanwhile, prices get pushed upward as the recipients of bureaucratic favoritism—those who've been able to game the system by acquiring a CON—gain relief from pesky consumer demands.

These features of American health-care are anything but new, but they represent intrusions into the marketplace that are, in principle, part of the same song and dance that is Obamacare. Indeed, the latter looms in the mind of Dr. Smith as a deliberate crescendo in the sneaky slide toward

---

5   For those wanting to read further on the less-than-saintly ways of many a nonprofit, I recommend a book by Harvard Business School professor Regina Herzlinger, *Who Killed Health Care? America's $2 Trillion Medical Problem—And the Consumer-Driven Cure* (New York: McGraw-Hill, 2007).

Single-Payer. He's not alone in thinking that the ACA is a willful attempt to destroy "from the inside" the workings of the free market—consolidating medical provision and alienating more and more consumers—in the expectation that the desperate masses will cry out to Washington for salvation.

But neither do these developments keep Dr. Smith from looking forward with optimism in the expectation that government meddling will unwittingly drive economical patients into the waiting arms of doctors prepared to have the consumer as judge. The optimism is underwritten, too, by his commitment to price transparency, effective management, and customer service. To show just how serious he and his colleagues are, since 2009 the Surgery Center of Oklahoma has posted its all-inclusive prices for procedures on its website—www.surgerycenter.com. As of January 6, 2015, to name a few examples, one can get a new pacemaker installed for $7,600, arthroscopic knee surgery for $3,740, or an inguinal hernia repair for $3,060.

The online pricing created what Dr. Smith calls "shock-waves," resulting in a much-needed deflation of surgery costs in places even quite distant from Oklahoma. The Canadians are a case in point. Shortly after placing prices on-line in 2009, Smith's Oklahoma outfit was greeted by a wave of our northern neighbors who would otherwise be advised to "hurry up and wait" in line for an operation. These were people "blessed" with Single-Payer coverage who were able to see the value in receiving timely, proficient care for a fraction of what other places were charging. Things have not let up for Dr. Smith and his colleagues in Oklahoma ever since.

DIRECTOR'S POSTSCRIPT

Another thing stood out when I reviewed the hours of footage I had of Jules and Keith Smith. Smiles. They both ooze a certain satisfying peace and happiness. I think part of that comes from delivering a valuable service to appreciative customers at an equitable price. This is one of the delights of capitalism.

So we at least know places to check in case we require personal care in Texas or surgery minus the hidden costs and heinous bills.[6] But what about

---

6   For cash-friendly doctors who are members of AAPS, go here: https://aaps.wufoo.com/reports/
    m5p6z0/.

the more general care for our bodies? What sort of considerations should be at work in our thinking and acting in regard to overall health? As we'll see in the next chapter, these are questions that deserve the attention of American Christians, especially at this time in our history.

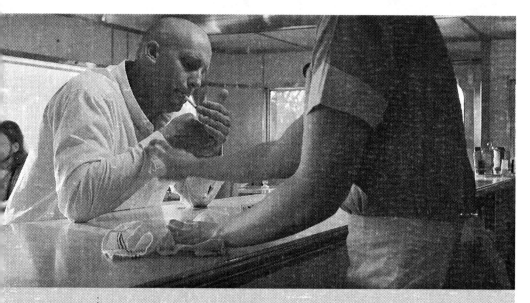

10 | A STEWARD OF ONE'S HEALTH

HONOR GOD WITH YOUR BODY

"Hello, My name is _____, and I'm obese."

How would you react if your pastor went before the congregation and to make such a confession? That's what Pastor Doug Anderson did not too long ago when he took the pulpit to bring the Word on a Sunday morning. He recently become convicted about the habits that led to his portly condition and was confronting both himself and the members of his congregation about their own participation in a popular Christian vice—gluttony. Confrontation (even when confronting oneself!) can be fruitful when it is done in a spirit of humility and is aimed at repentance. Judging from the fruit it brought, this was a case in point.

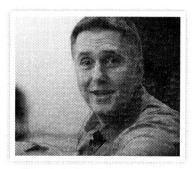

This is Pastor Doug Anderson, who was inspired to take his own personal health challenges before his entire congregation.

Thanks to a doctor who was unafraid to express concern for his patient and to the influence of a prominent Christian author on the subject of health, Pastor Anderson spent the months that followed the confession not only changing his own diet but also bringing his congregation through what they would later call a "transformation" of their mindset and lifestyle with respect to diet and health.

Of the many roots at the base of a flabby evangelical subculture, Pastor Anderson cites "stress eating" among church leaders who carry the weight of caring for the sheep. He also supposes that a Christian practice of feasting—otherwise good and commendable—provides opportunities for overindulgence in the name of fellowship. Yet a refusal to neglect the needs of the body or the Body should not translate to ingesting junk or allowing our bellies to be our gods. Having awakened to this, Doug sees more clearly now that a proper stewarding of the creation under Christ's lordship means using food and exercise for nourishment, not as a crutch. Even more pointedly for Christians, it means we must take responsibility before our savior as the delegated *custodians over and sharers of* a divine dwelling place:

> We eat comfort foods to bring us comfort. And I was convicted of that... because the Word of God says that the Holy Spirit is to be our peace and our comfort and that we are the *temple* of the Holy Spirit. So we started this series entitled "Transformation," where I challenged the entire congregation to follow me and to be transformed physically, emotionally, and spiritually... For me, the accountability was 1,200 people looking back at me every Sunday. And if I didn't follow through, I didn't know what was going to happen! So, I was *very* motivated to follow through.

In the face of what's been described as an obesity epidemic in the U.S., stories like this are encouraging. Though I view with scorn the effort of New York City's Mayor Bloomberg to regulate soda sizes, I also acknowledge that, in high numbers, Americans are suffering due to bad diet. Not only Americans but Christian Americans. in particular. It's been asserted that the Christian Church today suffers a "blind spot" in the area of caring for bodily health. Consider the study by sociologist Kenneth Ferraro of Purdue University, released in 2006, in which the author articulates that America's churches serve as a "feeding ground" for the country's obesity issues. Ferraro warns that, "if religious leaders and organizations neglect this issue, they will contribute to an epidemic that will cost the health-care system millions of dollars and reduce the quality of life for many parishioners."[1]

So, perhaps Mayor Bloomberg is properly motivated. He's aware that there's a scarcity of belt-buckle holes in America, especially in the Bible belt. All the same, I hope we can agree that Bloomberg's Orwellian tactics constitute an unhealthy response to an unhealthy people. What we need, especially within the Christian community, is *not interdiction but individuals* who will enjoy God's gifts responsibly, in moderation, with an eye to how they may bless the Church, and ever mindful of their witness to the world. Pastor Anderson agrees:

> There's a lot of talk about health *reform* and insurance *reform.* But I contend that we don't need reformation as much as we need transformation. We need to be transformed by the renewing of our minds and start thinking about health differently... Health is our responsibility. We can't depend on the *government* to keep us healthy or make us well. If we would just take care of our own bodies, as the Bible instructs us to, I think things would be a lot different.

He's seeking to practice what he preaches. By adding to his daily diet a gallon of water, a higher vegetable consumption, and a 45-minute walk, Doug succeeded in dropping 70 pounds within three months.

The author whose writings helped lead Pastor Anderson down that path and have continued to shape his thoughts and waistline is Dr. Scott Stoll. Dr. Stoll, who specializes in spine and sports medicine in Bethlehem, Pennsylvania, is influencing numerous Christians through materials like his book *Alive: A Physicians Biblical and Scientific Guide to Nutrition* (visit: http://www.fullyalivetoday.com).

I was thankful to interview Dr. Stoll and appreciated his proactive message. We can critique the mindset of those who are quick to bestow gratuitous medical costs on someone else. Yet, in our critique of such (which is well and good), if we don't also set to edify and maintain our own physical bodies, we become clanging, hypocritical cymbals. In the absence of physical fitness, we are, through our passivity, preparing to place burdens

---

1   Amy Patterson Neubert, "Study finds some faithful less likely to pass the plate," at https://news.uns.purdue.edu/html4ever/2006/060824.Ferraro.obesity.html; Internet; 2 August 2014.

on others. This may come in the form of transferring bills for heart operations or treatments for diabetes that arise from a lack of nutrition, but it may also come in less obvious, more subtle ways in which our testimony and usefulness as workers in God's kingdom sustains damage from ill-attention to our overall nutrition. I like what Dr. Stoll says about this, realizing as he does that staying healthy shouldn't be reduced to being concerned about what the scale reads:

> When I talk to people about their health, I really try to frame it in a way that they can understand that their health influences every area of their life... We think of health and *weight*... in reality, your health affects every relationship. It affects your work. It affects your ability to serve. It affects your ability to go on mission's trips. It affects the stewardship responsibility that God's given us... Your health is far more than just the weight that you see on the scale. Your health is the totality of your life.

It's refreshing that he is careful not to remove how we think of our physical life from the access and instruction of God. We are to walk before the Lord, loving him with heart, mind, soul, and strength.

Stoll is also aware, however, that Christians often mistakenly construe their spirituality in a way that places things of the Spirit in opposition to a debased world of matter.

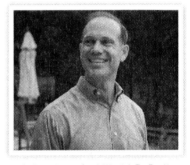

A physician and nutritionist, Dr. Scott Stoll guides people toward healthy eating and lifestyle. He's also a Christian with a clear message of responsibility and hope for the Christian community.

I'm referring to traces of ancient Gnosticism. Under such ideas, a supposed religious devotion can lead Christians to build islands of autonomy in their physical lives, one of which might relate to maintaining fitness. This is wrong. In what we call the Incarnation, the Son of God took to himself a body for the sake of redeeming his people, raising up their bodies, and renovating the cosmos. That reality at the center of Christian revelation and piety should be enough to send us in the right direction. Moreover, in reflecting on both the creative and re-creative character of God's works, Dr. Stoll reminds Christians of Paul's words in I Corinthians 6:19 and 20:

"You are not your own. You were bought with a price. There-fore, glorify God in your body and in your spirit, which are God's."... I think we've forgotten that as we go out into the world, we are ambassadors—to the world—of Jesus Christ. And the thing that people see, the first representation of Jesus Christ to the world is our body... We don't have to chase diets but by pursuing health our bodies naturally come to a normal weight. And then we can go forth... The beautiful thing is that people see our good works and glorify God who is heaven. And that should be the representation of Christ that people see, not a representation of conformity to the world.

Dr. Stoll is calling on us to eschew an imprudent conformity in the ways we feed and treat our bodies. This complements Pastor Anderson's emphasis on *transformation*, as opposed to the reactionary attempts by our politicians to bring *reformation* in the form of bureaucratically managed controls and regulations.

Something else of great importance in the first quote from Pastor Anderson relates to the matter of accountability. Part of being a respon-sible person involves placing ourselves before the judgment of others. We are prone to flatter ourselves, after all, lauding our own virtues and rationalizing our vices. I believe that this is so not only concerning what we stuff down our gullets but also—to return to a major theme of *Wait Till It's Free*—concerning how we handle our finances as they relate to health-care. Along these lines, I had an opportunity to speak with an entrepreneur who has purposed to improve the American diet by way of a "big box" health food store.

I'LL TAKE THE COMBO: HEALTHY LIVING AND CONSUMER SOVEREIGNTY

A few years back, a writer for the *New Yorker* characterized John Mackey as a "right wing hippie." The description seems pretty apt. The sixty-year-old CEO of Whole Foods evangelizes on behalf of vegetarianism (which he practices) while hiking cross-country. Then he'll throw you a curve by marketing meat, disdaining unionism, and espousing the free market principles of Milton Friedman. In their more generous moments, self-appointed "true believers" among the granola-eating crowd (who, sadly, too often are statists) will launch the rotten fruit of "sellout" and "capitalist," whereas Christians rightly raise skeptical eyebrows at the mystical atheism that nourishes Mackey's soul and wrongly frown on his selling of beer.

Yet along with the mixed reviews, the man some consider the Darth Vader of a health food empire has also brought a refreshing balance to the galactic conversation about health and health-care.

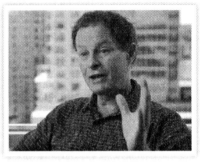

Having personally sat down with the paradoxical front man for Whole Foods, I've selected at least two features that stand out as strengths in his armor. First, consistent with the focus of this chapter, Mackey believes in front-loading the costs of health-care. That is, he grasps the need for us as individuals to invest in a nutrient-rich diet while understanding that so many of our sophisticated health-care efforts are reactionary measures taken late in the game:

A highly successful businessman, John Mackey believes in allowing markets to operate freely and insists on enjoying the fruit they produce.

> The great truth that's largely been ignored is that we *are responsible* for our own health... We eat incredibly bad diets in the United States... Sixty-nine percent of the adult population are overweight and a staggering 35% are now obese. We are... digging our own graves with our teeth... There's not going to be some kind of vaccination people give for cancer... and there's not going to be some pill you can take that reverses heart disease. It's going to be changing our diets and lifestyles. That is the *primary* solution to most of the health-care problems that face America.

Whether one embraces the sort of "whole food" menu that Mackey recommends or something closer to the "hunter/gatherer" (AKA paleo) diet, it especially behooves Christians to work toward minimizing the processed and empty calorie foods they consume. We may not be what we eat, as the saying goes, but whoever invented the saying at least recognized that dietary actions have health consequences.

Mackey has a keen awareness of this fact and as a businessman is not unmindful of the physical well-being of his employees:

> At Whole Foods Market... we do something called "total health immersions," where we put our sickest team members through a week-long dietary and lifestyle intensive educational program, with excellent food. And, literally, I've seen dozens and dozens and dozens of people lose over a hundred pounds of weight and keep it off in less than a year. I've seen type II diabetes reversed. I've seen heart disease reversed.

Along with such efforts to situate employees as the primary managers of their health, through diet and lifestyle, Mackey has also gained attention (both positive and negative) for seeking to engage his employees as sovereign consumers within the medical marketplace. This is what I perceive as a second robust feature of his armor.

In the U.S., we appear to be wedded—at least for the time being—to the notion that an employer is socially obligated to include some semblance of health-care provision as a component of employee compensation. Given this unnecessary but stubbornly persistent state of affairs, I think Mackey and Whole Foods go about equipping their employees to deal with catastrophic medical needs in a way commendably consistent with their pro-active approach to individual health.

For starters, Whole Foods offers its team members a high-deductible health plan (HDHP). This is a good thing on many levels. First, by combining lower premium payments with a steep initial cost to the beneficiary before claims will be paid out, the HDHP allows for and incentivizes greater savings. This is especially true for companies like Mackey's that pay into employee Health Savings Accounts (HSA), which allow unspent contributions to roll over year to year. It also, arguably, encourages the beneficiary to maintain good health and to act as a savvy consumer, seeing as most of us would rather spend time and money on enjoying life than having tests and procedures done only because "we have the technology" (with apologies to the six million dollar man). Along similar lines, the HDHP designates the consumer-patient as payer of the "first dollar" toward medical care, discouraging the over-consumption and soaring costs associated with high premium plans or a "fed as first dollar payer" approach.

In this vein, a virtue of HDHPs is that they represent a welcome departure from the dysfunctional system of prepaid health insurance. Mackey offers some insight:

> The whole point of insurance is... you want the insurance to kick in if you get cancer or you have a car accident. Well, obviously, you're not going to be able to... easily... go out and compare prices for that. But that's where I think insurance plays a valuable role. Similarly, when you have automobile insurance, which is very competitive... in prices, the insurance company isn't paying for your oil change... tune-ups... new tires. You pay if you have an *automobile accident*. In health-care we've got it reversed. They think that health-care should pay for *maintenance*, when, in fact, it should only pay... when truly something horrible happens to you... You should be protected, so that you don't have to go bankrupt, you're not financially ruined.

In other words, he's of the school of thought that insurance should function as *insurance*. It should not serve as an enabler of economic laziness. It should serve as a prudent recognition that we are finite and vulnerable; insurance premiums are monetary markers of that fact. Things happen to us that are beyond our control. Events can overtake us that we didn't and (often) couldn't anticipate or avoid. To stretch insurance beyond its appropriate role as a catastrophic backstop, in Mackey's judgment, may as well lead to the absurdity of having something called "grocery insurance." No need to estimate whether that block of cheese is reasonably priced. Just show 'em your grocery insurance card. But if that seems nuts (or cheesy!) to us, then why have we for so long failed to see the absurdity of such buck-passing in the realm of health-care provision?

At least a partial answer to this question consists in the fact that we have, as a society, become less directly accountable to each other and to local institutions (such as family and the Church). Instead, we have transferred our accountability, along with the burden of providing a social "safety net," to centralized institutions and programs. In doing so, we have not only robbed ourselves of an important component of Christian compassion but also removed critical supply-and-demand signals from the marketplace. Without operating in terms of a Christian understanding *per se*, the

Whole Foods collective is attempting to resist the centralizing trend by empowering individuals to direct and finance their health-care costs.

In its presumptuousness, however, a creature such as the Affordable Care Act is not only lessening Mackey's ability to bless employees in that way but also undermining his ability to run a competitive business:

> We're being forced to cover many things that we used to not cover before—mental health or alcoholism... adults up to 26 years of age on their parents' plan (they may not be dependents anymore). There are all types of things that are raising our costs. There is no free lunch. So, as costs go up, we... pass those on to the team members at large by raising deductibles or raising the premium cost or doing what many businesses are doing, which is lowering the number of full-time workers that we have.

Indeed, at the time I interviewed him the percentage of full-time Whole Foods team members was set to drop from around 75% of its workforce in 2013 to 70% of its workforce in 2014.

At the risk of sounding like a broken record, these are the sorts of un-intended socio-economic ripple effects that we can expect to see as the State garners a greater portion of the health-care market through myriad mandates and regulations. We thus have reason to be quite disappointed and concerned about the direction we're headed—which includes an entitlement-minded culture, stymied creativity and innovation, and curtailed economic freedom. Nonetheless, as I've said, there are reasons for liberty-minded people to have an optimistic outlook.

KARIS: PATIENTS AND PRICES

One institution whose people are working on behalf of consumer-patients—namely, by achieving discounts on medical bills—is The Karis Group (https://thekarisgroup.com). Tony Dale accidentally started Karis about twenty years ago. It really was an accident, too. Contrary to my view that British people shouldn't play basketball, Dale, a former NHS doctor, was contending with his kids on the court when he injured one of his knees:

> I was fairly aware that I had torn my medial collateral ligament. So I went to see an orthopedic surgeon and he confirmed what

had happened by MRI and told me it would take about $2,000 to fix it… But because I came from another country… I didn't understand the system. And so $14,000 in medical bills later… for about a half an hour of work… I had to find a way to pay all those bills. I wanted to understand what was happening in the system. And that's when I challenged the bills and, to my amazement, everybody was more than willing to negotiate the bills. Out of that grew this idea that most people out there would not have the courage to negotiate their own bills and maybe we could help them.

Under Dale's direction since 1996, Karis gives patients an audible voice within the complex and sometimes intimidating world of medical billing. The key, he says, is to be bilingual:

What we do… is we see a problem and we step in. The problem is that patients and doctors or patients and billing departments or patients and insurance companies don't know how to talk to each other in the same language. We speak both languages and we're able to bring them together and bring them to a place of agreement.

A primary goal of this sort of patient advocacy is to prevent the injured or sick person from having her body repaired at the cost of a broken bank account or credit rating:

From our point of view, we're not just dealing with a number. Hospital billing departments, your typical medical practice, a radiology clinic—they're handling hundreds or even thousands of these cases. They don't… think of themselves as dealing with people. So, when we reach out to them and say, "Oh but do you know anything about Mrs. Smith? How much has already been paid by the insurance company? What proportion of this are you expecting to come out of her pocket?" In that context, it's very easy for us to personalize… and that we need to find a win-win. A win-win isn't the hospital necessarily getting all of its money. And a win-win is certainly not the patient walking away not paying for valuable services. A win-win is finding a fair and appropriate price.

Such efforts to negotiate have become a practical necessity, as over the past two decades increasing numbers of people find they are unable to afford pre-paid medical (or much of it, anyway). Additionally, as consumer-friendly care is now set to dissipate further due to new levels of government meddling, the burden of charge master rates and various rationing devices (in the form of waiting lines or flat denial of care) is also set to be even more heavily placed upon the backs of those with little or no insurance coverage.

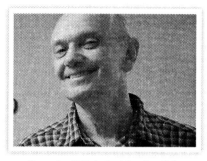

Formerly a British physician, Tony Dale founded The Karis Group, a collection of patient advocates who negotiate medical bills for cash-pay patients.

Clearly, therefore, Karis is providing a valuable and powerful service. That being said, Dale's own agenda is driven by more than a desire to accomplish cost saving. As a person who is very familiar with the challenges posed by the health-care industry and who is also a Christian, he is eager to talk about an approach to health-care financing that is both effective and in line with an ancient biblical teaching and practice. I call it the Samaritan approach.

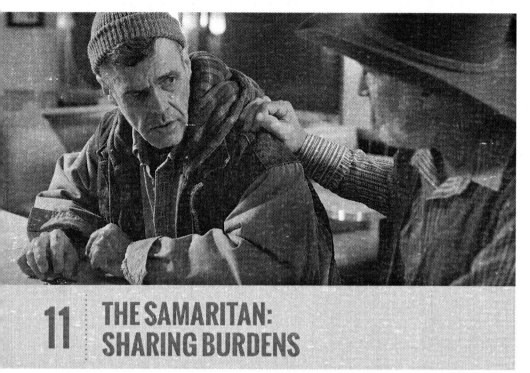

11 THE SAMARITAN: SHARING BURDENS

OUR CONFESSION AND ITS IMPLICATIONS

From the outset, it's been our intention in this book to focus on *the body*. How could a book claiming to be centered on patient care, after all, not have such a focus?

As a general starting point, allow me to reiterate the Christian affirmation that the Triune God is Lord of *this* world. We believe in the Creator of heaven and *earth*. He did not form the soil and seas in order to turn his attention and concerns exclusively toward ghosts and immaterial beings. In acknowledgement of Adam's historical body and the consequences of his fall in calendar time, God sent His Son *in the flesh*.

Moreover, those benefitting from the Son's humble walk upon the earth both with and for them have not been left to an esoteric spirituality. Rather, the Lord is pleased to employ humble, earthen vessels in the forgiving and healing of those who were sick and guilty. Spiritual men in local assemblies are charged with keeping watch over our sheepish souls. As those in union with the Christ who conquered sin and death, we live with the hope of the resurrection, a Spirit-provided embodiment *after* life after death. As such, our lives should be lived in light of God's creative, redeeming power to renew us, in our totality, along with the rest of creation.

It's against this backdrop that I hope we will view the plight of patients. A Christian philosophy of medicine and health-care must balance God's affirmation of the *goodness* of creation with the acknowledgement that its present state is one of *groaning*. Likewise, we ought to weigh on one side a grateful confidence about the understanding we have of the body and the instruments we have to sustain and repair it, and on the other side the humble admission that we are limited in what we can do and that our true hope is in God. Our attitude should be in line with the words of Shadrach, Meshach, and Abednego when they told Nebuchadnezzar:

> If we are thrown into the blazing furnace, the god we serve is able to deliver us from it, and he will deliver us from Your Majesty's hand. But even if he does not, we want you to know, Your Majesty, that we will not serve your gods or worship the image of gold you have set up.[1]

We don't take for granted the breath of life. But we also hold it with an open hand, trusting the wise and benevolent providence of our Savior.

PATIENTS AS MEMBERS OF CHRIST'S BODY

In the opening stories about Roger Stuber, Claudia Swanson, and their families, my emphasis was on the plight of the patient. We may be equipped with all the drugs and instrumentation the world has to offer, but if we allow these or the interests of other parties to crowd out a central concern for physicians and their patients, then we have become addicted to the pricey life-flight helicopters and many other fancy accoutrements, possibly leaving health-care behind.

What I only touched on in the first chapter, however, and wish to explore a bit further here, relates to the peculiar way in which the Stubers and Swansons paid their bills. How did they stare down the barrel of the often outlandish and intimidating world of medical billing and live to tell about it? How did they, without taking State-aid or buying an insurance policy (which, contrary to a Christian's best wishes, is likely to involve their payments going toward things such as abortifacient birth control pills), come out relatively unscathed from their respective brushes with heroic medicine and the extreme price tags attached to it?

---

1   Daniel 3: 17, 18

From a financial standpoint, they were able to do it because each of these families had earlier joined a health-care sharing group called Samaritan Ministries. But it's important to stress that taking "the way of the Samaritan" involves much more than a financial standpoint. As we've already said, it involves a crucial confession of faith and, with that, a commitment to supporting and caring for the community of believers.

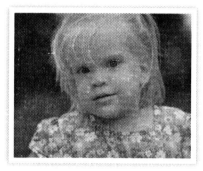

Samaritan Ministries members came alongside her parents and paid Claudia Swanson's medical bills.

In the story of the Samaritan, found in Luke 10:25-37, Jesus instructs his listeners that the man who, without any other religious credentials to his name, loves his neighbor is the one who rescued and tended to a beaten stranger and paid for the man's care, even to his own hurt. In Galatians 6:10, Paul's exhortation to the churches is to "bear each other's burdens, and so fulfill the Law of Christ," doing good to everyone, "especially those of the household of faith." It was then, by the power of the Spirit, that the early Church drew together, as we read in Acts 4:

> Now the full number of those who believed were of one heart and soul, and no one said that any of the things that belonged to him was his own, but they had everything in common. And with great power the apostles were giving their testimony to the resurrection of the Lord Jesus, and great grace was upon them all. There was not a needy person among them, for as many as were owners of lands or houses sold them and brought the proceeds of what was sold and laid it at the apostles' feet, and it was distributed to each as any had need.[2]

Communism, you see, is not a bad idea. The Acts church is a case in point. These saints demonstrated true charity by voluntarily sharing their resources among the household of faith.

Is biblical communism allowed anymore, though? Haven't we just talked about how the new lawless law of the land requires us to either have

---

2   Acts 4:32-35.

insurance, be a welfare recipient, or pay a fine? As it turns out, that's not entirely true. The Affordable Care Act, for all its heinous cronyism and humanistic adoration of State power, contains at least one decent portion. Tony Dale, founder of the Karis group, was eager to encourage Christians by sharing about an exemption that, by God's grace, made its way into the ACA's pages:

> You know, to every cloud there may be a silver lining. And one of the things I actually love about the Affordable Care Act is that tucked away in those thousands of pages that we wouldn't know till it was passed was actually a provision for Christians, if they chose to live Christianly.

What he's referring to is 26 United States Code Section 5000A, (d), (2), (B), an exemption to the requirement that individuals and their dependents maintain an essential minimal coverage or pay penalties:

> (B) Health care sharing ministry
> (i) In general, such term shall not include any individual for any month if such individual is a member of a health care sharing ministry for the month.[3]

Not only does Samaritan Ministries meet the criteria laid down in the exemption, but people within the organization's leadership played a significant role in lobbying to include the exemption in the law. Thus, the ACA law itself does not prevent Christians from escaping, as it were, into a health-care sharing ministry.

The headquarters of Samaritan Ministries International (SMI) is located in Peoria, Illinois, only a two and a half hour drive south of the city of Chicago. In the fall of 2013, our crew traveled there to learn more about SMI's history and what makes the organization tick.

As a member of Samaritan Ministries, I had the privilege during that visit to meet the founder and president of SMI, Ted Pittenger. Pittenger, who launched Samaritan Ministries as a non-profit in 1994, using as a base of operations an 11' by 15' portion of a former chicken coop in his backyard, summarized how this type of cost-sharing works:

---

3   Copied and pasted from: http://www.law.cornell.edu/uscode/text/26/5000A; Internet; 2 August 2014.

Samaritan Ministries is not an insurance company. But we provide an alternative to insurance for a way to meet one another's medical needs... And we do this on an organized basis. Some people may think we're just gonna pass the hat and hope that we're going to help one another... but it's organized, it's computerized... We talk in terms of member households. And a household might be a family of any size, it might be a couple with no children, and it might be just a single person. Each one of those categories constitutes a household that shares a particular amount each month. They can count on that... so they can budget for that. It's just a matter of us telling them where to share that money each month. So each month we send out a newsletter, where they have the opportunity to share in another member's need. And they would send that money directly to that person to help with that particular medical need.

The staff here acts as a clearinghouse to take the needs, makes sure they fit our criteria, and then divides up those needs to be shared by our members.

At the time of the interview, Samaritan allocated around $6 million in need sharing every month. In less than a year, however, the membership added around 10,000 households (and counting), and the need sharing is now up over $10 million a month.

Yet a distinguishing feature of Samaritan's model of *direct* healthcare sharing among Christians is that it offers a much more intimate connection on the financial end of things

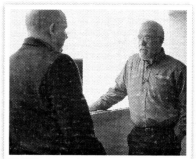

I spoke with Ted Pittenger, founder and president of Samaritan Ministries International, a direct sharing ministry in which Christians join together to meet one another's health-care expenses.

than an insurance policy or a Medicare payment. Members not only exchange monetary gifts to meet needs, but they are also asked to send notes of encouragement and offer up prayers on behalf of those who are suffering various maladies and receiving medical treatment. The same can be expected from members of the SMI staff, who frequently pray with and counsel members who call in with inquiries or requests.

This reliance on prayer shows that, although the staff is constantly in communication with members and helping them as they interact with health-care providers, there is a strong organizational insistence that God is the all-sufficient Provider. Alongside this emphasis, the Samaritan Guidelines, which establish expectations of members and explain the process of having needs "published," carefully direct Christians to local sources of support (family, church) as their initial "emergency response team" in the face of sickness, disease, disorder, or injury. While the guidelines do technically permit Samaritan member funds to be used as a supplement to State-aid, insurance, or both, the ministry largely seeks to reorient the thinking and language of its members away from a prevalent *consumer* mentality and feeling of entitlement. As a society, we are completely saturated in language and concepts native to insurance (not to mention the subtle trappings of benefitting from coercive wealth transfers), so it's easy to fall into a certain mindless "insuranceSpeak"—even for those endeavoring to take a distinctly non-insurance route to health-care financing.

Insurance, after all, involves a transfer of risk from the insured party to the insurer. This accounts for why one speaks of insurance "claims." The nature of the agreement between the insured and the insurer is such that the insured has a claim on the insurer, with respect to the terms of their policy agreement. Now, there's nothing wrong with that as such, but it's a different animal from direct health-care sharing. Direct health-care sharing operates through the avenue of voluntary, non-contractual giving. As such, a member seeking to have needs published and shared retains 100% responsibility for supplying the need processors with itemized bills and for supplying payment to the provider. On the flipside, the confidence placed in the sharing members, does not take the form of a claim a member in need has on the dollars of her fellow members. Rather, the confidence takes the form of a grateful, mutual reliance among members of a shared faith community. In the same way that someone might leave a church, those who come to take lightly the mutual reliance within the sharing network by withholding shares are dropped from membership after a time if they fail to mend their ways.

It's refreshingly clear that, for the Samaritan leadership and staff, need sharing is not just a job, but an adventure. As Executive Vice President of

SMI, James Lansberry is well aware that direct health-care sharing is not a model of pristine efficiency. But that's part of the point. Samaritan is not about offering a slick, modified insurance model; it's about offering a very different kind of approach and experience altogether:

> Our members are in a community with one another. Because of that they are not just getting the bills paid by some faceless insurance company. They get checks and notes and cards, and that encouragement... is just an amazing piece of the puzzle. And I'll just tell you a little about my own experience... this year. We just had a baby... his name's E.J. He was born in January, but he was born dead. He had no heartbeat when he was born. And they resuscitated him, and he spent eleven days in NICU, which is just an amazing expense. Our total bills... altogether... totaled over $200 thousand, which I don't carry around in my pocket and I bet you don't either. And so, we're trying to engage in that cost picture... So I see those bills... and I negotiate with the hospital, with the doctors to try to get something a little closer to a fair rate.

> But that $200 thousand means that I had hundreds of families from around the country—that I'll never meet—sharing in that burden with me... I've got a stack in my office of cards six inches high... from 42 different states, [people] who are praying for us, taking the time to share with us, taking the time to pray for E.J. and his health. And so it's an amazing experience. It's much different than you'd ever see from an insurance company because it's personal.

That experience of personal support and accountability also, as he mentions, plays a key part in re-engaging individual patients and consumers who are involved in exchanging dollars for goods and services.

One way that Samaritan particularly seeks to re-engage its members as savvy, frugal health-care consumers is through what's known as the Standard Need Reduction. For any bills a member submits for publication after calling in and "starting a need," the first $300 in charges is not marked to publish. That initial amount falls exclusively to the member requesting support. In practice, that up-front reduction of what is allocated for members to share actually functions like a classic deductible. Essentially, it serves to discourage hasty or excessive consumption and, at the same time, requires a considerable "buy in" on the part of those incurring bills. The practice of "patient dollar first" also has an overall effect of encouraging Samaritan members to take a pro-active approach to their health, to prefer healthy eating, and to engage in regular exercise.

An additional exciting feature of the Standard Need Reduction makes it quite different from a regular deductible. Although it serves a good economic purpose, a deductible is pretty much an unqualified discouragement for the patient-payer. What's different about the Standard Need Reduction is that any discounts a member can obtain on their original bill totals count dollar-for-dollar against the initial unpublishable amount. Members are thereby encouraged to "earn" the unpublishable amount, saving themselves and often the other members, by entering the medical marketplace like they might a car dealership (i.e., skeptical of sticker prices). This benefits members by adjusting their monthly share costs in a downward direction. It also places a positive pressure on the suppliers of health-care services to offer more or better services while still operating within the world of voluntary exchange. Of course, when we talk about the overall economic benefits achieved by an intimate network of mutually supportive cash-pay patient-members, we're talking about a few rocks causing ripples in a massive lake. A few ripples, however, are better than none.

A CALL TO ACT ON BEHALF OF QUALITY, AFFORDABLE CARE

So, if you're a Christian and you're not yet disillusioned about the common ways we do health-care financing in this country, then you must first become disillusioned. Once you've done that, go looking for an alternative that is self-consciously Christ-honoring. When you go looking, at least consider Samaritan, and ask yourself why you'd hesitate to join a community of this sort that's seeking to very practically and consistently care for the body of Christ here on earth. James Lansberry would exhort you to reflect on your Christian values and make a decision in line with those values:

> One of the additional reasons why Christians ought to be looking at organizations like Samaritan for their health-care is that whole unequally yoked principle... We pray for pro-life principles, we pray for pro-life politicians, we pray that God

would end the scourge of abortion and then we subsidize it through our health insurance dollars... But trying to look for a health-care option which is consistent with your religious values is important. And in the age of Obamacare, in the age of the Affordable Care Act, we've only exacerbated that. Right now, any insurance policy, starting in October [2013] has to cover Plan B, the so-called abortion pill, the so-called emergency contraceptive. So *any* insurance plan that you participate in covers that emergency contraceptive, which we consider to be antithetical to the pro-life principles.

Being a part of something that is, like Samaritan Ministries, consistent with your Christian values, with your pro-life values, is even more important than... getting the need met. It also allows you to express your Christianity in that transaction. When Jesus talks about holding every thought captive, through Paul, every thought captive to Jesus Christ, what we need to be thinking about is how we think about our health transactions in a way that holds those thoughts captive to Jesus Christ... "Look out not only for your own interests but also the interests of others... bear one another's burdens and so fulfill the Law of Christ."

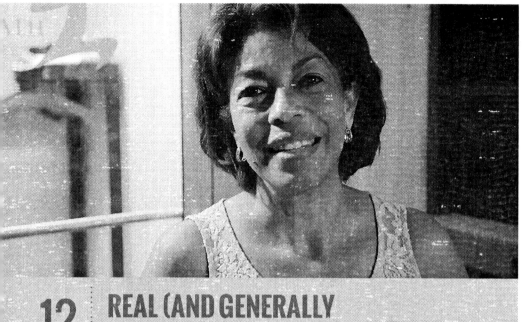

12 REAL (AND GENERALLY AFFORDABLE) CARE ACTS

WORKS OF CHARITY

It should be clear by now that our call here for a return to health-care liberty is not part of a social Darwinist program. It is not, for example, congenial to the atheistic ethics of someone like Ayn Rand. We are, after all, seeking to emulate the mindset and attitude of the Samaritan, sacrificially carrying each other's burdens and, at least partly as a result of carrying those burdens, properly reaping the blessings of health and wealth that the Lord will grant through our love for one another. Yet this shouldn't tempt Christians to thumb our noses at the world from within the safety of a tidy, spiritual bubble.

As Christ's disciples, we are to wash each other's feet. Certainly, strong Christian communities are vital expressions of the power of the gospel and the unity of the Body, but if we're not careful, this mindset can mutate into an all too comfortable circling of the wagons. At no point in the story of the Good Samaritan, however, does the unexpected protagonist pause to confirm the bruised man's religious credentials before deciding to help. What I mean to say is that there should be an outward flow of our desire to practice tangible, from-the-heart charity. Those outside the household of faith—strangers to the covenants—should see our good deeds, experience at least the earthly benefits of them, and glorify our heavenly Father because of them.

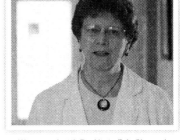

The work of Dr. Alieta Eck gives us a glimpse of the kind of mindset and enterprise that I'm trying to encourage. Some time back, Dr. Eck, partnering with her husband, also an MD, opened Zarephath Health Clinic, a charitable medical clinic located in Zarephath, New Jersey.

We visited with Dr. Alieta Eck. She and her husband, Dr. John Eck, run a charitable clinic in Zarephath, New Jersey.

Dr. Eck does not mince words in saying what she thinks of so-called government charity. When I provoked her by playfully suggesting that it's the government's job to care for the poor, she kindly countered:

> The government cannot really provide medical care for the poor. All it can do is meddle and coerce and restrict and under-pay for what it's promising to give to the patients.

I later asked what she thought of socialized medicine and what it entails, giving her opportunity to discuss the consequences of State involvement more generally:

> The government, when it gets involved in medical care, has to set up guidelines. And they have papers to be filled out to find out if people qualify because people might try to game the system and get on when they're really not eligible. So, constantly they're coming up with rules and they call it fraud and abuse when people get on when they shouldn't be. And it's a constant pressure to keep costs down. So, you have people that enroll, the State runs out of money, and then they can't find physicians. And everybody's frustrated. Taxpayers are just being fleeced. So, when socialized medicine happens, it always runs into shortages. There's always an infinite demand for medical care when it's "free."

Dr. Eck has experienced these realities not just from the comfort of an armchair.

In 2003, she and her husband opened their charitable health clinic, largely motivated by their experiences of the waste, clutter, and inefficiencies accompanying state-financed care:

> The reason we started it was that the Medicaid system was so laden with paperwork and bureaucracy that we would spend money filling in the forms and by the time we got paid the doctor got nothing... and still had to pay all the overhead. So, we decided if we were going to care for the poor—and we didn't want to abandon the poor—we would set up a clinic apart from our private practice and have all volunteers and... private donations pay the bills. And it wound up being a very, very good model.

This decision permitted their staff of donors and volunteers to bless people who are struggling and also to cultivate a spirit of charity among the recipients:

> As the economy has gotten more and more difficult, and people lose their jobs... We have students who get out of school with debt, and they can't find jobs... There are always gonna be people who are stuck... They just don't have the money... And usually that's just a temporary state to be in. We help them when they need it, and then they get back on their feet and they get their jobs. And then they'll come, and they'll donate time or money to help us. So, it's a nice cycle. And anybody, at some point or another, could find themselves in a place where they need help.

Her observation about the category "poor" as not some permanent, monolithic group of people is also insightful. Those properly perceived as poor are sometimes those who've been knocked over by disruptive or tragic events. People lose their jobs and experience hard times. This does not mean that they are necessarily accustomed and acclimated to an impoverished *way of life*.

Regardless, Dr. Eck views her efforts as the privileged duty of a Christian to care for her neighbor:

> We have a brochure that we give out to patients that tells the story of the Good Samaritan. And it explains the concept of one individual seeing that a person's in need and *personally* meeting that need. He put the patient on his own donkey... and paid... and the patient got well. And the patient was enriched by the situation and the Good Samaritan has been immortalized because of it. And notice he didn't look for a government program to help that poor person. He just said, "I can do it, I'm gonna help, and I can take care of the person in need."

I believe that Dr. Eck is expressing in her professional ministry as a physician an attitude and an understanding that all Christians should possess. We have each been blessed with gifts, talents, and resources. And it should be viewed as our privilege to put those toward not only serving our own interests but also the interests of others.

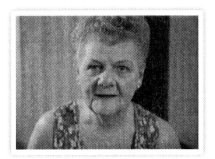

"Praise the Lord!" The gratitude from all of the patients was obvious.

PICKING UP MEDICARE'S TAB

As part of our call to be wise stewards of our resources and to associate with the broken and hurting, we also have an important obligation to care for our elderly. Sadly, however, we commonly have the attitude that serving our parents is *someone else's duty rather than our own joyful privilege.* This way of thinking and feeling, of course, makes a certain kind of sense when you stand back and look at our political situation and the ideas that have shaped it.

Medicare did not appear *ex nihilo* from a puff of Stalinist smoke. It came along gradually and we accepted it. You reap what you sow. What was sown was a socializing of elderly care most prominently through the apparatus of Medicare (in a way strikingly similar to the socializing of child-care through the machinery of government schooling). The catch is that, with only a little oiling, machines tend to work on their own once they're up and running. The machine need only be built, switched on, and occasionally reformed.

As we pondered in the film, a chugging momentum in the direction of socialized health-care was something that Ronald Reagan understood and warned our parents and grandparents about in 1961. With him, the organizers of Operation Coffee Cup saw the writing scrawled on the wall of the diner stall. In the days of vinyl records, they made an effort to "go viral" with the message. In those days, what this meant is that the wives of some AMA doctors got together and campaigned against socialized medicine.

Of course, for the Christian, a fundamental objection to coercive redistribution of scarce resources relates to the fact that the latter requires a progressive deconstruction of property rights, as well as the nuclear family.[1] That objection, it turns out, has not proved to be a historical winner over the past fifty years. While proceeding down the track Reagan warned about, we Americans pull behind us an endless line of boxcars loaded with the familial and financial ruins we've accumulated.

From here, we've got to move a bit deeper to address our current malaise.

There are, no doubt, multiple complex issues relating to our attitudes these days toward those who are 65 and older. I don't wish to oversimplify these matters, but it's apparent that not only the perpetuation of the Welfare State but also the economic depression the U.S. has suffered since 2008 have, together, generated "social friction" between Baby Boomers and their successors. Fleshed out a little more thoroughly, one reason for this friction is that the bankruptcy of Social Security and Medicare is hitting home for a generation of young taxpayers. Even bleeding heart undergrads, after all, are apt to get upset when they learn that unfunded liabilities for these statutory mandates exceed $100 trillion. Sprinkle on top of that sad sundae the fact that our Central Bank is printing over $60 billion every

---

1   For a recent defense of private property, see Shawn Ritenour, http://blog.tifwe.org/private-property-and-human-flourishing/; Institute for Faith, Work, and Economics; Internet; 8 October 2014.

month in order to suppress interest rates and pump a stock market that no longer functions based on fundamentals.[2]

More pedestrian statistics can be just as dismaying to those graduating with a ton of student loan debt into an abysmal job market. These would include the observation that, as far back as 1999, those 65 and older spent nearly five times per capita on health-care as people under 65. When those numbers are placed in a context in which able workers are serving as the unwitting benefactors (AKA tax slaves) of their elders while being told that the "trust fund" won't be there for them, at least a little of what the French call *ressentiment* is understandable.

Nevertheless, as those who are in Christ, we are not bound to such generational tensions and, indeed, must transcend them. In view of the fact that, in Christ there is now neither "Jew nor Greek, neither male nor female," it's a reasonable inference that neither are there old nor young. We are all one in Christ. There is still, however, an economy and an order of things. Within the framework of God's economy, children are commanded to honor their parents, the first commandment with a promise, "that it may go well with you and that you may live long in the land." James announces that "pure and undefiled religion before God" is marked by caring for orphans and widows, those usually least able to sustain themselves and make ends meet. Furthermore, in Proverbs 20:29, King Solomon declares: "The splendor of old men is their gray hair." We are to preserve a dignified and respected place within our social intercourse and economic planning for those who are getting on in years, especially our own kin. This is God's opinion, which automatically qualifies it as warranted and true.

We're not here talking about patronizing the elderly. Too much of that happens in our society as it is. Too many octogenarians, for example, are babied and made to feel at home with the idea that they are physically and mentally beyond contributing wisdom or reasonable service to the community. What we're talking about here, rather, is cultivating close personal connections with and a willingness to financially support our own parents and other elderly, especially those who are members of Christ's body.

Exemplifying this spirit in the film were David and Carol Bridges, and their family. About five years ago, it became quite evident that Carol's mom

---

2   "Stocks recover losses, close up nearly 2% on Fed minutes," http://www.cnbc.com/id/102070077; Internet; 8 October 2014.

was not thriving in the large house she'd live in alone for years. Her memory was failing, she wasn't eating as healthy as she used to, and she was not coping well with the responsibility of managing the property and finances. The challenges were mounting. It was then that a sibling pow-wow was called. Through that meeting, a decision was made that grandma would come and live with her daughter and her husband. Somehow, Carol says, she had always known her mom would end up coming to stay with them.

She was eager to welcome her mom into their house and home. Indeed, many good things came out of that decision that would likely not have materialized if Carol and her siblings turned their mother over to the professional care of strangers. One important outcome was that, by living with the Bridges, grandma has been able to transition gradually into living as a dependent without feeling emotionally toppled by suddenly being treated as a helpless patient. This has had different facets to it.

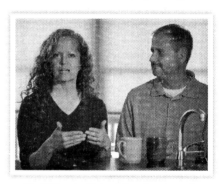

First, by coming back into the family setting, grandma is not isolated. She plays an active role in her family's life. She's been able to read to the grandchildren and be the listening grandmother. This

The Bridges family has taken steps to repair and cultivate an important relationship with an elderly relative.

has had the positive impact of allowing Carol some rest on the parenting front. The presence of grandma also helps the children to realize that the world does not revolve around them. In grandma, they have some "friendly competition" for the kind attention they naturally expect from mom, dad, and even their siblings. Grandma is permitted, therefore, to retain a dynamic dignity and not suffer the uncharitable assumption that she is an invalid just because she's old.

Along with the "social benefits" afforded by grandma's presence, the Bridges' home has arguably provided an environment more geared to nurturing grandma's individual wholeness and well being than a more clinical care-giving facility might offer. *Wait Till It's Free* obviously places a great deal of emphasis on removing impediments to the relationship between the givers and receivers of medical care, but it's not a foregone conclusion that a nursing facility, say, will help grandma see her present condition (e.g., in which she suffers the effects of dementia) as part of a whole, meaningful life. Without disparaging nurses as a class, we can appreciate what it means for Carol to have her mom around and vice versa.

For Carol, personally, there've been blessings. For example, she tells about having light shed on previously obscure or altogether unknown aspects of her mom's (and thus her own) life. Moreover, the nurturing of their relationship enabled Carol to help her mom understand things that happened to her even many years ago but which she may not have processed well in the intervening years. For example, the Bridges cite the fact that she's been forced in some ways to confront, rather than suppress, the memory of her husband's death over three decades ago, and as a result, she's been able to grieve that loss in a healthy way.

Regarding her physical health, the Bridges have been able to manage grandma's care proactively. Being quite familiar with her health history, they largely have a sense of what she needs. They also have a sense of what she prefers. For instance, they point out that her resistance to medical interventions is more likely to encounter a sympathetic ear in their home than it would in a clinical facility, where her attendants would be more likely to medicate by default. In line with the philosophy of Whole Foods CEO, John Mackey, the Bridges frontload their "medical" expenses by focusing on a healthy, organic diet, drinking plenty of water, and staying reasonably fit through exercise. As such, they take a proactive approach to their family's health management, and grandma is an important part of the family.

Let's not fool ourselves. There's no solving or saving the insolvent programs of Social Security and Medicare. Thank the Lord for that. Other than Hell, all bad things must come to an end. What this means, however, is that, other things being equal, people with fixed incomes—many of whom rely on these programs—can expect, in coming decades, to see their dollars lose purchasing power and their standards of living suffer. What it also means is that we increasingly face the choice to either reform our ideas about the proper function of individual, familial, ecclesiastical, and civil governments according to the standard of Scripture or suffer the civilization-eroding consequences of refusing to reform. I'm hopeful that, by grace, we will choose the first of these two options.

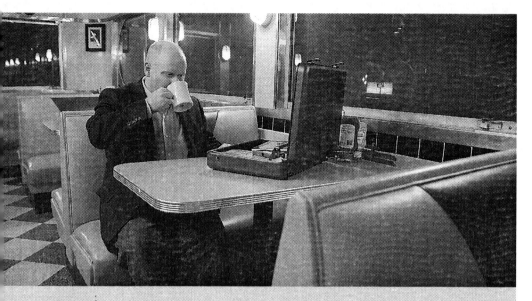

13 NEW REWARDS

COUNTING THE COSTS OF CARE

Toward the end of our film, we surprised a few people by showing the arrival of my newborn son, Theodore Livingstone Gunn.[1] Theodore was born right at the end of the post-production stage, a very busy time, and is recorded taking some of his first breaths in the final moments of *Wait Till It's Free*. The story of his arrival, I felt, had relevance for our project on multiple levels. At the least, Theodore's presence in the film helps draw attention to the fact that these are not merely academic economic concerns that we are addressing in the realm of health-care. Related to the very personal nature of a baby birth are the very personal details (yes, some of which are "economic"—from the Greek *house law*) of how that baby birth plays out.

Along these lines, I can confidently say that, from our family's stand-point, nothing over the past several years more plainly reflects and affects our attitudes about the health-care biz than Emily's childbirth experiences. But in unpacking that statement, I first want to drive home a bit of philo-sophical common sense. Let it sink in that a person's ideas about what the *problems* are in the world (which will sometimes bring him into conflict

---

1   It might interest some readers to know that we named him after Theodore Beza, the Reformer who succeeded Calvin in Geneva, and David Livingstone, the Scottish missionary from the area in Scotland called Lanarkshire, where I'm from.

with those who see things differently) will be determined by his *beliefs and preferences* about how the world should be (often in contrast to how the world *is*). As an illustration, when I've accompanied my wife to hospital births, my moral and economic scruples have, increasingly, led us to be very selective about which hospital services we deem necessary or beneficial.

If the reader will recall both my Scottishness and the fact that I'm a member of the Samaritan Ministries share network, it should be understandable why the force field already surrounding my wallet suddenly magnifies when I enter a hospital. But seriously, when you detach from the cold embrace of an insurance policy, thereby assuming 100% legal responsibility for your medical bills as well as the responsibility of stewarding the volunteered dollars of others within the share network, you should expect to become more thoughtful about the value and cost of the goods and services being offered. You should become aware of and generally more conscientious about your consumption habits. The simple fact of price awareness should be enough to steer you away from the easy path of thoughtless consumption and her devilish twins, increased scarcity and price inflation. In short, you should transform into an ordinary and yet powerful cost-benefit analyst. Shorter still, you should become a functioning market participant.

I have very vivid memories from our last birth at a hospital a few years ago. I was serving as the custodian of the community's resources that day. That's no joke. Because I was paying cash, I had the audacity to view our use of the hospital's services as a collection of economic exchanges at arm's length between two parties (*us* and whichever hospital worker happened along, offering to provide some good or service). Every physician and technician that entered the room met with questions about the cost of the services they were aiming to deliver. Poor folks! And more than a few skilled medical professionals were politely shooed away if we thought we could reasonably do without what they were "selling" or could provide it ourselves for a much lower price (lower, for example, than $200 for a Vitamin K shot or $250 for a hearing test).[2]

---

2   Hospital staff members, by the way, are just as likely as patients to be clueless about the costs of medical goods and services. Perhaps even more odd and ironic is that a nurse's annoyance at the price-consciousness of a savvy cash-payer is really an annoyance at the sort of attitude that someone is likely to have who appreciates the value of good service. Humans generally rank the value of something purchased in terms of what they are willing to give up in order to possess it, but it can be emotionally difficult to be subjected to the free market choices of someone within an environment that's, in many ways, shielded from such blatant economizing on the part of local, individual consumers.

Unfortunately, my cost-consciousness also ran up against the depersonalized nature of what too often passes for health-*care*. Our system may train people to know about maintaining or improving health in some respects, but in that middle space between (if not altogether surrounding) doctors and patients—the space occupied by insurers and hospital conglomerates— some of the *care* gets lost or, at least, stymied. In our experiences, this reality shows itself not only in the form of bitter nurses and patronizing OB/GYNs but also in the annoyance of hospital staff members when we dare to ask about the price of something or show any propensity to haggle.

It wasn't until we started filming *Wait Till It's Free* that I was able to make better sense of why cash-paying patients frequently feel the same way Russian restaurant patrons felt before the collapse of Soviet communism. Within our third-party payer health-care system, you are viewed more as a *consumer* of time and resources than as a *customer* worthy of quality service. A nuisance.

As a rule of thumb, the consumer exercises considerably less sovereignty in attracting the help of a supplier once the bill has been paid in full. This is because health-care coverage providers (HMOs, insurers) largely operate on the assumption that, since they already have been paid for seeing

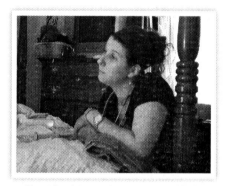

We paid cash to a midwife, who treated Emily like a valued client.

you, they are inclined to see you as little as possible. This does not mean that all those working within a system dominated by third-party payers who charge hefty premiums mean to neglect or stiff the patients. It does mean, however, that those individual servants who choose to make it all about patient needs are swimming against a system that places the interests of corporate financiers in competition with the interests and well-being of patients.

He who pays the piper calls the tune. What this proverb means for prospective patients is that, when they forego closely directing and financing their own health-care, they permit (nay, invite) those on the stage (doctors, technicians, nurses) to play to the wishes of other parties.

My wife and I have found that doing home births is one way for us to pay the piper, but instead of paying a piper (who I wouldn't be inclined to trust delivering a baby), we pay a midwife. Not only, however, does this not mean *marrying* the midwife, it doesn't even mean, for me, being married to the idea of doing home births. It's certainly preferable to have ready access to emergency services should they be necessary. This can indeed be achieved in most cases of a home birth, but there are important reasons for choosing to do a home birth these days, even in addition to the advantage, as comedian Jim Gaffigan puts it, of not having one's wife give birth while dressed in a gown someone may have died in yesterday.[3]

As a cash-paying home birther, you are fully engaged in the cost picture. Instead of paying for a $25 aspirin, washed down using a $5 paper cup and walked over to us for a small fee of $35, we most recently purchased all of Emily's birth supplies on Amazon (which, if you have Prime, adds no shipping costs!). It's fairly typical to be billed $2-5 thousand for a home birth. That amounts to paying somewhere between $\frac{1}{10}$ and $\frac{1}{2}$ of what one would face for a standard, trouble-free hospital birth.

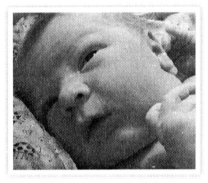

Introducing our ninth child, Theodore Livingstone Gunn

In exchange, if you're blessed as we've been, you'll find a great midwife. The midwife we last hired remained on call and clearly loved providing the services we required. She takes what I consider the healthy view that childbirth is not properly thought of as a medical problem and liability to her and some massive clinic that employs her. We were her employers and, as such, we assumed most of the liability. As our resident professional, she prayerfully trusted in God's wise providence to see mother and child through the labor and delivery.

Along with the many economic thoughts and lessons it points us toward, however, Theodore's birth also underscores a theme of new birth

---

3 Gaffigan also parodies home-birth skeptics as saying: "Oh yeah, we thought about doing a home birth but we decided we wanted our baby to live." He jokes, of course, as one whose wife had all five of their children in the comfort of their two-bedroom, New York City apartment. See Jim Gaffigan, *Dad is Fat* (New York: Crown Publishing Group, 2013).

and renewal that worked its way into *Wait Till It's Free*. The title of this chapter is "New Rewards," taken from a phrase Samaritan Ministries uses to announce the birth of a child, but there are other sorts of new rewards that we learned about in making the film. I'm thinking here of people who experienced the benefits of taking greater responsibility for their health through improved diet and exercise.

In an earlier chapter, I discussed how Pastor Doug Anderson confronted issues of gluttony in his own life and in the church and how he was blessed by the work of Dr. Scott Stoll. When we went to meet with Dr. Stoll, he paid us the additional benefit of inviting another of his student-patients to come and visit. That created what turned out to be a highlight interview for us. It was our Natalie moment.

Natalie is a slim, slightly shy woman of Italian decent. She has a broad, appealing, New Jersey accent. She smiles and sighs when discussing her fondness for Italian food—with an emphasis on the bread and pastas. Natalie went on to share openly how her untamed appetite led to a severe weight gain over a number of years, eventually placing her life in danger. She told us how she managed to eat her way into a Rascal scooter, one of those little vehicles commonly seen trundling the morbidly obese around stores. Eventually, she even outgrew the scooter, so that when she climbed aboard, the Rascal wouldn't move.

Having reached a health crisis point, Natalie began consulting with doctors. She did not receive much hope from them apart from recommendations that she have gastric bypass surgery. That's how things went before she met Dr. Stoll, whose optimism and direction led her to take drastic but appropriate (and non-surgical) action. As mentioned, Natalie had dwelt on a carbo-centric, American-Italian diet (the kind that rivals guns and knives for its ability to dispatch well-rounded mobsters like Tony Soprano). What Dr. Stoll did was train her into a completely new mindset and diet. Through his instruction and exhortation, Natalie moved onto a plant-based diet and the results were profound and inspirational.

In the film, we document the amount of weight she lost, but I don't want to focus so much on the pounds. Instead, I want us to think about the rebirth that Natalie experienced in her life. Due to the leading of a gracious helper and her own willingness to forsake complacency and embrace a responsible, grateful attitude toward her health and the body

God's given her, she embodies a lot of the lessons I hope people will take away from *Wait Till It's Free*. Natalie's *life* has been changed. As we briefly chronicle in the movie, by turning her back on a life of obesity and severe dependency, she was able to see her *body* redeemed. In the process, she was able to return to communing with the local Body of Christ. She now fits into the pews and has the opportunity to reconnect with the preaching of the Word of God and to enjoy the mutual support and encouragement of the Church.

This directs us back to some of the big themes we've been talking about in several previous chapters. The Lord has seen fit not to make us sprightly spirits. He made us, instead, living and breathing body-souls. We are earthen vessels, not ghosts trapped in physical prisons. As such, we are to act as responsible stewards of our health, loving the Triune God here on earth with all our heart, mind, soul, and strength.

But this can't be just a formal theological lesson that we store in our brains, as I've come to appreciate. Indeed, two very traumatic and unexpected things happened to me personally through the making of the film and the writing of this book: diet and exercise. In the chapter about the UK, we talked about some of the moral hazard that gets promoted (wittingly or not) when statist efforts and taxpayer funds are made to subsidize unhealthy lifestyles.

Truthfully though, I've had some owning up to do with respect to my own conscience as a Scotsman who, by definition, enjoys hearty food and drink. It can be difficult to explain the routines of Scottish pub life to the average Southern Baptist.

It's not just my Scottishness that's to blame, of course, for the... well-rounded shape my body's had for the past several years. I'm also a bit of a computer geek. This means that I do a lot of sitting around. If I'm working, that, at least often, means I'm at my desk. If I'm working hard, I'm probably at my desk even more.

But I'm done making excuses.

I make the point at the end of the film that I cannot very credibly preach about health responsibility while being nonchalant with my own health and fitness. Along these lines, consider that other famous documentary filmmaker I mention in the film. Rivaled only by his hypocritically large bank account (in view of his complaints against capitalism) is the vast waistline of Michael Moore to which viewers of the health-care documentary *Sicko* are treated. The image of his sizable silhouette served as a, perhaps, superficial but nonetheless real motivator for me to step up my game when it comes to health management. I thus resolved not to be just another chunkified "American health-care crisis" documentarian. One, I think we can agree, is enough.

Thankfully, I've found other, more substantive motivators for trimming down and taking better care of myself. It hasn't *all* been about one-upping Michael Moore or doing a plump Colin/trim Colin scene for the movie. In particular, reflection on my role as a husband figured largely (no pun intended) in my recent turn toward improved fitness. As I was forced by my own film to think things through, I realized that a wife and mother—notably my own wife and the mother of our children, Emily—lays a lot on the line physically to produce and sustain a family. When I think of Emily it strikes me that she has made considerable sacrifices in her own physical comfort, strength, and even health to bear multiple children and manage a growing household. In light of this, I as her husband became convicted about my hypocritical attitude.

Not only am I a husband. I'm a father. It's important for dads to be fit and capable. We are called to serve the family, not so much ourselves. I'm also a churchman, a public representative of Christ. If I'm okay with being obese, don't I risk placing a stumbling block before those rightly inclined to view with some suspicion a fat prophet? Having big responsibilities shouldn't serve as an excuse for being too big for one's britches. I've thus realized that I must personally own the message of personal responsibility that we present in this book. This realization helps to account for why I found myself wearing a trash bag and jogging in the rain at midnight on my 40th birthday.

A CALL TO ACTION

Let me, then, exhort the reader to think well and long about your responsibility before God to steward the resources he provides. He gave you a body to care for and, if you're a spouse or a parent, he's given you more than one. He also gave you the ability to work, to plan, to invest, and to build for the sake of God's glory as well as your neighbor's benefit.

With these thoughts in mind, I exhort you to commit to taking greater responsibility for managing your own health. This should involve taking a pro-active approach to *edifying* your own body, both in what you eat and drink as well as the activities you agree to participate in. It should also involve taking a pro-active approach to financing your own health-care. If you are thinking of visiting the State-subsidized exchanges, for example, instead think about visiting here: http://www.healthcaresharing.org.

If you are a Christian, then you are called to serve Christ by taking up your cross and following him. Part of what that means is that Christians are to be known as people who are not eager to have their neighbors, much less perfect strangers, foot the bill for their own consumer demands. On the other hand, to reiterate a theme from the Samaritan chapter, we read Paul's instruction in Galatians 6:10, that those in the churches are not only to be committed to bearing their own burdens but also to *volunteering* to bear the burdens of others, in particular the burdens of those among the household of faith. In seeking to apply these insights, those in Christ should desire to share their own resources and be willing to receive assistance from their fellow saints when sickness, injuries, and the price of body repairs threaten the livelihood and prosperity of an individual or family.

With an eye, then, to our mutual responsibility to uplift our brothers and sisters in the Lord, let us diligently lighten those burdens, realizing that quality medical services are a scarce economic resource. Unless you're the Creator, you can't get something for nothing. One way we can lighten the load is to become savvy market participants. By becoming more aware of the price of quality care and by working to economize wisely within our own households, we will help bring greater price transparency and improved customer service to the medical marketplace. In doing so, we will also bless our Christian siblings by allowing them to put their material resources toward other, constructive Kingdom work.

Another facet of the message set forth in this book relates to the importance of seeking out and establishing relationships with sound, caring medical professionals. This, of course, rests on the assumption that there are sound, caring medical professionals to be found. As we show in our film, such creatures do indeed exist. My encouragement and exhortation here is that now, more than ever, we are a country in need of doctors who will heed the call, take seriously their role as agents of healing, and put the good of their patients before all other professional loyalties.

The healing of the healing profession in the U.S. will take place only when the doctor-patient relationship is restored to the honorable status it was given by Hippocrates, but for this to take place, the *doctor* part of the equation and its restored integrity is paramount. *If you are a medical professional,* learn from the principled stand taken by numerous physicians in our film. Pursue excellence in your field, serve the patient with diligence, don't get diverted into a quest for riches, do works of charity, be committed to free market medicine, fiercely resist government intrusion into healthcare, and don't let yourself be bribed or co-opted by the expanding reach of bureaucratic bloat or the manipulative tentacles of crony capitalism. Uncover and expose the forces of tyranny and corruption where you meet them and, above all, stand for the sanctity of human life.

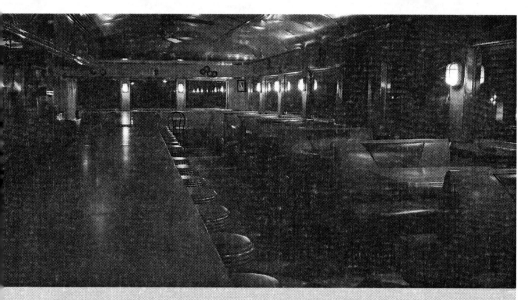

POSTSCRIPT:
A CONCLUSION AND A PREDICTION

On a parting note, let me say that I hold to an *optimistic eschatology*. By that I mean that we should have high expectations for what the Spirit of God is doing in the earth. Concretely, we should look forward to God's powerful grace converting people in droves as well as to a bursting forth of the fruit of the Spirit in calendar time. Not all Christians, of course, agree with me in this view. Nevertheless, it is important to distinguish the belief that the knowledge of Christ will someday cover the earth the way the oceans do from specific political hopes and expectations we have. One can see the future as bright in terms of God's unfolding plan of redemption (akin to a mustard seed that grows up into a tree upon which the birds come and rest) without assuming that the spiritual and ethical wisdom of the Bible is soon to be promoted at the ballot box.

In light of this, what we should be after, as the prime mover of any political action, is for the Word of God to inform all areas of our thought and action. This requires us to take an *incrementalist* approach that's focused on communicating biblically derived thoughts. By reaching hearts and minds, our Christian duty should include intellectually re-shaping the social, economic, and political landscape of God's world.

Having produced *IndoctriNation*, I often, in discussing the matters raised in that film, reference a revolution that took place over the past half century in the realm of education. The revolution took the form of a widespread rejection of government schooling. Driven in many quarters by conscientious Christians, a distinct cultural division occurred, resulting in what came to be known as the Christian schooling and home-schooling movements. In the face of a growing secularism in the land and led by outspoken advocates for private alternatives, Christians voiced a demand for such alternatives and were met by increased supply (as evidence of this, find a home-schooling convention in your area to attend). Bottom line: the move toward Christian schooling and home-schooling is largely a grassroots phenomenon, spearheaded by purposeful activism. Yet, for all that—and here's the rub—successes in the direction of politically or legislatively deconstructing the machinery of government schooling have been slim to none (and slim left town last week).

What's my point? My point is that a similar, grassroots revolution—or perhaps better, *reformation*—needs to take place first in our hearts and minds with respect to how we *think* and *do* health-care. What would the future of health-care and health-care financing look like were such a reformation to take place? I believe we could expect to see results comparable to the evident fruit produced (and still being produced) in those places where Christian schools and home-schooling cropped up. If Christians will deliberately, thoughtfully join forces, form cohesive communities, and share the burden of each other's medical expenses while storming the gates of Heaven with prayer, the Christian community will increasingly embody the spirit of voluntary love and support that characterized the church we read about in Acts.

As a corollary to that reality, dependence upon government and even on third-party insurance coverage will gradually fade as the light of Christian responsibility and charity shines forth. I believe the results of such a development will be manifold, including a healthier Christian community, the restoration of price sanity, and both the improvement and increased availability of top-of-the-line medical goods and services. At the same time, I expect that, as Christians "clean house" among themselves, government-run health-care will take a decidedly different trajectory, sliding heavily in the direction of rationed care and less serviceable facilities. Simply put, American health-care will increasingly come to resemble Britain's National Health Service.

Now, isn't that reason enough to resist slouching toward socialism?

Under such worsened conditions, one at least hopes that even overt enemies of Jesus will have the sense to admit that the religion of Statist Interventionism produces yucky fruit. Regardless, rather than passively dawdling down the messy path to socialized medicine, I choose to heed the proponents of a better way, many of whom are featured in the preceding pages. I hope you will, too.

INDEX